FINDING
YOUR
VOICE

Brian W. Hands
MD, FRCS(C)

FINDING YOUR VOICE

A Voice Doctor's
Holistic Guide
for Voice Users,
Teachers, and
Therapists

Published in 2009 by
BPS Books
Toronto, Canada
www.bpsbooks.net
A division of
Bastian Publishing Services Ltd.

ISBN 978-1-926645-06-3

Cataloguing in Publication date available
from Library and Archives Canada.

Cover illustration: Jeffrey Hands
Text design and typesetting: Tannice Goddard, Soul Oasis Networking

Printed by Lightning Source, Tennessee. Lightning Source paper,
as used in this book, does not come from endangered old growth
forests or forests of exceptional conservation value. It is acid free,
lignin free, and meets all ANSI standards for archival-quality paper.
The print-on-demand process used to produce this book protects
the environment by printing only the number of copies that are
purchased.

*To my wife, Cynthia, and my sons, Jeffrey and Stuart,
whose voices have soothed me and helped me
through these many years.*

*And to the memory of my mother and father:
Without their "voice" I would not be here.*

CONTENTS

Preface   ix

Acknowledgments   xv

Introduction   1

I THE VOICE
1 Voice Production 101   9
2 Energy 101   25

II THE DISORDERED VOICE
3 A Visit to the Voice Doctor   43
4 The Most Common Vocal Problem: Muscular   54
   Tension Dysphonia
5 Other Vocal Problems: The Results of   61
   Abuse and Misuse

III THE ORDERED VOICE

6 Vocal Communication: The Fifth Chakra   69

7 Vocal Support: The Third Chakra   76

8 Vocal Artistry: The Fourth Chakra   82

9 Vocal Stance: The First Chakra   85

10 Vocal Creativity: The Second Chakra   89

11 Vocal Intuition: The Sixth Chakra   92

12 Vocal Spirituality: The Seventh Chakra   94

13 The Wear, Tear, and Care of the Voice   97

Appendix: 109
The Gag Reflex as an Indicator of Muscular
Tension Dysphonia

References   115

Atlas of Vocal Disorders   117

Glossary of General Terms   123

Contents

Preface   ix

Acknowledgments   xv

Introduction   1

I THE VOICE
1   Voice Production 101   9
2   Energy 101   25

II THE DISORDERED VOICE
3   A Visit to the Voice Doctor   43
4   The Most Common Vocal Problem: Muscular   54
    Tension Dysphonia
5   Other Vocal Problems: The Results of   61
    Abuse and Misuse

III THE ORDERED VOICE

6 Vocal Communication: The Fifth Chakra   69

7 Vocal Support: The Third Chakra   76

8 Vocal Artistry: The Fourth Chakra   82

9 Vocal Stance: The First Chakra   85

10 Vocal Creativity: The Second Chakra   89

11 Vocal Intuition: The Sixth Chakra   92

12 Vocal Spirituality: The Seventh Chakra   94

13 The Wear, Tear, and Care of the Voice   97

Appendix: 109
The Gag Reflex as an Indicator of Muscular
Tension Dysphonia

References   115

Atlas of Vocal Disorders   117

Glossary of General Terms   123

PREFACE

My purpose in writing this book is to give voice to my work, knowledge, experience, and passion for the benefit of professional and amateur voice users who are suffering with vocal problems or wish to prevent them. This group includes singers, actors, teachers, professors, broadcasters, lawyers, executives, auctioneers — anyone who uses their voice in any manner for the communication of art, information, or ideas. I have written it as well for those who work with voice users, including voice teachers, voice coaches, and speech-language pathologists.

I used the word *passion* above because it describes my own involvement in this work. Indeed, I feel blessed to have helped voice users of all types, including actors and singers, for more than three decades. I am still surprised and am always thankful that my journey has led me to such an exciting and fulfilling career. I hope readers will indulge me a brief description of that journey, though it does bear directly on the content of this book.

It began when I was in grade five. Singing in the Glee Club was the major social event for boys and girls in my school in Toronto. As far as I was concerned, failing to get into this choir would make me a social outcast. Twenty-nine of us arrived for the audition: fifteen boys and fourteen girls. The music teacher, aware of the effect that rejection would have on us, let all of us join. However, he quickly figured out that I and four other boys could not sing. What to do?

In the case of one song, "My Grandfather's Clock," he found a way to save our face — and the audience's ears. Our role was not to sing but to cluck with our tongues against our cheeks, mimicking the sound of a clock ticking. That was it.

This music teacher is a friend and a patient of mine all these many years later, and we often laugh about my auspicious, if not suspicious, beginnings. He is fond of saying, "Brian, I knew you would be successful in your career, but I never thought it would have anything to do with singing."

I received my medical degree and my specialization in otolaryngology (the ear, nose, and throat specialty) from the University of Toronto. As part of my residency, I took a year of surgical training in San Francisco. I was in a study club during that time, which met in the home of one of my professors, the Chief of Otolaryngology at the University of California, San Francisco. We discussed the physiology of the voice and also took some field trips to the San Francisco Opera.

I loved music but had not been exposed to opera except through listening to LP recordings.

My first opera concert was scintillating, thrilling, and awe-inspiring. Live theater plus music plus great stories sung in a way that felt so personal, moving, and intimate — it was like a movie spectacular, only bigger, better, grander, and more real. I was hooked.

I became fascinated by the voice, this musical instrument that can produce pure sound without the modification of tubes, chambers, valves, or stops — the purest sound a human can make.

I completed my residency in otolaryngology after my fellowship examinations in ear, nose, and throat. I then joined the Central Hospital, Toronto, which had been founded by two Hungarian doctors — John and Paul Rekai — after they fled their country following the Hungarian Revolution in 1956. One brother was a specialist in internal medicine; the other was a general surgeon.

It so happened that the internist — Dr. Paul, as he was affectionately called — was a passionate and knowledgeable lover of opera. He sat on the board of the Canadian Opera Company. Not long after I took up my clinical responsibilities at the hospital, he called me in to his office.

"You will be the doctor for the opera company," he announced in his thick accent.

I was flattered, intrigued, and concerned. I felt I was well trained and capable; however, I was keenly aware that I had not been prepared to care for the professional voice. On a scale of 1 to 10, my residency training in vocal problems was 0.1. I knew what vocal cords should look like but knew nothing of voice-production pedagogy and precious little about opera and its demands on the voice. My musical training was limited to a year or two of piano back in the mists of time.

I could easily make clinical diagnoses regarding the status of patients in my office or even in the operating room. But determining the status of a professional voice, deciding how to treat it, and knowing whether or not it was safe for a singer to sing that night? All this was too lofty for me. I knew that vocal careers are made or lost by decisions such as these.

However, despite my qualms, I decided to proceed in this new direction. I enrolled in extra training courses, consisting primarily of seminars in the United States. I served on panel discussions at international symposia. I studied in New York City with one of the great voice specialists of all time, Dr. Wilbur Gould. Once a month, for four months, I flew to the Big Apple on a Thursday and spent part of that day and all of Friday in his office. (Fridays began with breakfast at 7 a.m. at the Carlyle Hotel at 76th Street and Madison Avenue.) Dr. Gould was the voice doctor for Broadway productions and the Metropolitan Opera. As I grew comfortable with him, I grew comfortable with myself and my own abilities. I also spent time in Philadelphia with Dr. Robert T. Sataloff, a professor of otolaryngology and voice specialist at Thomas Jefferson University.

As theater burgeoned in Toronto during the late 1970s and 1980s, courtesy of productions by Livent and Mirvish, more and more Broadway-bound shows previewed in the city, with the great performers being cast in the major roles. *Cats* got it started, and then along came *Phantom of the Opera*, *Show Boat*, *Ragtime*, *Chorus Line*, and *Les Misérables*.

Performers often needed help with their voices as a result of colds and vocal strain. The company managers and producers would call the Canadian Opera Company and ask for the opera's voice doctor. "So and so is ill and tonight's the preview," they would say to me. "You've got to get these people to sing, Brian. I've got millions riding on this show. You've got to fix their voices."

I also became involved with the Hollywood movie companies whose stars were filming in Toronto, a.k.a. Hollywood

North. And rock concert producers would call before a big show with similar stories of woe. They too told me of singers whose voices were failing. The show venues were big: Exhibition Stadium, Maple Leaf Gardens, the SkyDome, the Air Canada Centre, Roy Thomson Hall, Massey Hall.

My services were also used by the Stratford Shakespeare Festival and several major recording studios, including Capitol/EMI, Sony Music, and Warner/Universal.

As this aspect of my clinical practice grew, I began downsizing my conventional ear and nose work. The voice became the major — and most enjoyable and exciting — part of my career. In fact, in 1996 I established a professional voice clinic called Vox Cura — Voice Care Specialists. It was at the time — and still is — the only free-standing, non-hospital-affiliated practice of its type in Canada, dedicated to the care and treatment of the professional voice. This center gives access twenty-four hours a day and seven days a week primarily to amateur and professional voice users. It is one of the busiest diagnostic and treatment facilities in the country.

I work closely with my colleague Aaron J. Low, a kind, understanding, experienced man who is really more of a voice specialist than his title of speech-language pathologist would suggest. Aaron is an invaluable part of the voice clinic. He is adept in fiberoptic endoscopy and videostroboscopy (technologies for examining the throat and vocal cords). He has taught me a lot during the years we have worked together. Anything beyond the medical scope of treatment in our practice relies on his unique expertise and abilities in understanding breathing and vocal resonance techniques, and most importantly in knowing how to release a patient's voice muscles and associated neck muscles while applying changes to incorrect voice behavior. Also helping me at the clinic is Steven

Henrikson, a vocal coach who was chair of vocal studies at the University of Windsor and who sings and teaches opera and Broadway singing.

I have been privileged to meet and work with some truly talented people, though I confess that sometimes I am not perfectly up to date on the big singing stars out there, as the following story illustrates.

Once, about eight or nine years ago, my secretary informed me that Aerosmith was coming in to see me.

"I don't know who Aerosmith is," I said.

"You know," she laughed, "the big rock group."

"Oh," I said.

At the appropriate hour the lead singer of this group entered the clinic with his entourage of driver, bodyguards, and producer.

I came into the waiting room and said, "Mr. Smith?"

There was no response.

"Aero?"

Fortunately Steven Tyler saw the humor in this exchange, giving me a smile and a laugh.

Whatever the style or genre of the actors and singers I treat, the greatest "high" I experience is to see them perform onstage, or in film, or in a play and know that I have played a small role in giving pleasure to the audience that night.

ACKNOWLEDGMENTS

I am grateful to the many people who have helped me — personally and professionally — in my medical practice and in writing this book.

Earlier in my life I was influenced by my grade-school and high-school teachers who got me organized to study. I fondly recall moments with my grade-five homeroom teacher, Mr. Burrows, and my grade-six homeroom teacher, Mr. Williamson, who kindly and thoughtfully taught me how to read and learn.

I'll never forget my English teacher, Miss Ford, and my Latin teacher, Miss Toll, both of whom guided my enthusiastic, creative thoughts, helping me transcribe them into readable English. I recall Mr. Bill Featherston, my grade-eight homeroom and English teacher, who introduced me to the Romantic poets Keats, Shelley, and Wordsworth. Through him

I realized for the first time the incredible beauty and power that words can hold.

My medical career was supported by professors Arnold Noyek and Jacob Friedberg, both of the University of Toronto Medical School's Department of Otolaryngology. Their knowledge, insight, and experience helped shape me into a more compassionate practitioner. Both are still practicing ear, nose, and throat specialists.

Instrumental in challenging me to write a book was my rabbi, Dow Marmur, who taught me the three pillars of a fulfilled life as set out in the Jewish Talmudic text *Pirkei Avot*: teaching a student, planting a tree, and writing a book. I am grateful, with the publication of this book, to have completed the third pillar. As for the other two, I taught first-year medical students in the University of Toronto Medical School's Department of Anatomy and lectured on voice to theater students at Ryerson, and I became a graduate landscape designer, after taking night classes for five years at Ryerson.

Dr. Howard Book, a man of great insight and clinical and professional experience, has served as my mentor. Dr. William Cass, a man always filled with wisdom and sensitivity, has been my dearest friend and teacher. He very kindly helped me by editing parts of this book.

Al Forest, P. Eng., my friend and cycling partner, gave me encouragement and spiritual counsel throughout this project.

In addition to all these, I wish to acknowledge Barb Semenick, Barbara Moses, and Annie Jacobsen — and every voice user, professional or otherwise, who has brought me challenges, surprises, and excitement with each visit.

Most of all, I want to thank my wife, Cynthia, my "college sweetheart" and best friend. Her love inspires me, her joy lifts my spirits, her wisdom and insight bless me, and her bound-less energy and zest for life keep me going. If I had only you by my side, *dayenu*, this would be enough. But you have also given me two sons, Jeffrey and Stuart, of whom I could not be prouder. Thank you, Cynthia. Thank you, boys. I love you each so much.

INTRODUCTION

As a medical doctor, I am trained to concentrate on my patients' physical symptoms and problems. I have found, however, that to treat these properly, I must consider more than their vocal and breathing "apparatus" and their medical symptoms and conditions; I must also take into account their emotional and spiritual concerns. If voice production involves the whole person, then whatever goes wrong in a patient's life — and hence with their psyche — will affect their body and their voice.

This makes sense. Voice problems are not isolated to disease in the throat or the larynx or "voice box" areas. In fact, most of the patients I see in my office rarely turn out to have disease of the vocal cords from disordered anatomy. Their difficulties are almost always caused by the compensatory actions they have taken to create sound when they cannot use their voice fully or do not understand how to use it properly.

These actions — for example, trying to "muscle" their sound with the muscles of their neck and throat, instead of breathing with the powerhouse of the diaphragm and supporting their sound with their abdominal muscles — are generally caused by stress and insufficient breath support. This tends to have a deeper source elsewhere in the body, which in turn has been affected by anxiety and stress — and on it goes.

I believe that every aspect of one's self-care, lifestyle, and emotional environment matters in vocal health: what one eats and drinks; how one sits, walks, and sleeps; and even how one thinks. All of these factors have an impact on the voice, so much so that they can actually shut it down. If something is wrong at any point in this system, the voice can fatigue easily and become pinched, strained, or uncomfortable. Not only will this affect the quality of the tone produced, it could lead to a chronic voice disorder.

To heal a voice, I cannot just look down a patient's throat for something red and swollen and prescribe a pill. Coaching is required as every aspect of the patient's health and lifestyle is examined and discussed until the body's entire system is functioning fully and energy is flowing freely through the body and out through the voice.

The voice is a "mirror of the soul." It reflects a person's emotional and physical state. An ordered, harmonious voice reveals an ordered and harmonious mind and soul. A disordered voice signals the practitioner to seek the cause behind the defective mechanism involved.

Many voice users feel that their instrument is a mystery, something only their teachers, coaches, speech-language pathologists, or physicians can help them with when they are experiencing vocal difficulties. *Finding Your Voice* will help such readers understand the mystery and take charge of their own voice. While the book does not contain vocal exercises or voice coaching, it will illuminate how the voice is integrated into the mind, body, and spirit. It will help voice users be active participants in the preventative measures they may need to make or treatment options they may need to take.

It is important for me to acknowledge here that the science of voice physiology is constantly being researched, evaluated, and redefined by my colleagues and mentors. This book does not attempt to synthesize or encompass every finding and every type of approach. It focuses, rather, on what I have learned during my practice as I have helped patients feel less in the dark. However, though I do not deal with vocal technique in great detail, much of what I discuss may help voice users with their technique.

In summary, this book, as the title puts it, is a voice doctor's holistic guide to caring for the voice. It is based on a view of the human body as a complete functioning system capable of producing beautiful art (or effective communication, or good work) through the instrument of the voice.

Here is how I address these issues.

I begin, in Part I, The Voice, with two chapters on the basics of voice production:

— Chapter 1 is an introduction to the anatomy and physiology of the human vocal apparatus: the physical processes by which organs and muscles vibrate the vocal folds (cords) and produce sound.
— Chapter 2 looks at the body as an energy system. This approach will be familiar to those who have practiced yoga or certain martial arts or who are familiar with

Eastern philosophy and medicine. I have found these schools of thought to be a useful framework for studying the body as a living, dynamic energy system. This chapter touches on the seven chakras, or energy systems, of the body, and how they relate to the voice.

What I have to say about these energy systems comes from Eastern traditions that go back nearly five thousand years — teachings that are increasingly supported by new medical research. However, it is of no great matter whether the chakra system is taken literally or metaphorically. Either way, understanding the system can be revealing for those working to protect and project their voice. (And let me add that this holistic approach to otolaryngology — the part of medicine that deals with diseases and disorders affecting the ear, nose, and throat — is now being practiced by a growing number of voice doctors and therapists, notably in New York City and Philadelphia.)

Part II, The Disordered Voice, examines the most common problems voice users experience, whether from abusing or misusing their voice. The three chapters in this part of the book look at how these problems are caused, as well as at their symptoms, signs, and proper treatments.

Part III, The Ordered Voice, goes more deeply into holistic care of the voice. Each of the seven chapters focuses on an energy center (chakra) and how it pertains to the voice user's overall health and the way the voice functions.

The book closes with a chapter that discusses lifestyle factors, including diet and exercise, to help voice users protect and care for their voice over the years to come.

Throughout the learning journey of this book, I will

illustrate various points by sharing some behind-the-scenes stories from my practice.

My aim and hope is that readers — whether they are amateur or professional voice users, or work with voice users as a therapist, coach, or teacher — will find this book of assistance emotionally, spiritually, and physically: in short, that it will help them find their voice.

PART I

THE VOICE

CHAPTER 1

Voice Production 101

Talking is so natural to us (*too* natural, for some of us) that we rarely think about how our voice actually works. However, a basic understanding of the structure of the voice will pay handsome dividends to voice users, as this chapter's quick tour of the basics of vocal production will show.

The Structure of the Vocal Tract

The voice-production system is made up of four parts

1) the *generator*, or diaphragm and lungs and abdominal wall
2) the *vibrator*, or vocal cords (a.k.a. vocal folds; the terms are interchangeable)

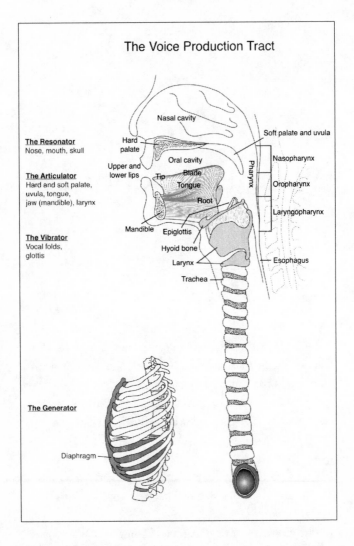

The Voice Production Tract

3) the *resonator*, or the space between the vocal cords and
   the top of the nose (tongue, palate, cheek, lips, and jaw)
4) the *articulator*, or the space where the sound comes out:
   the nose, the mouth, and the head.

The generator

The most important member of the four-member vocal tract is the generator, or the diaphragm. Why? Because the diaphragm is the key to proper breathing and (along with the

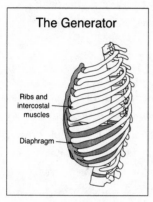

The Generator

Ribs and
intercostal
muscles

Diaphragm

abdominal muscles) breath support. Without breath, there is no sound. When we take a breath, two actions occur: The ribs are pulled out horizontally and the diaphragm drops vertically. The diaphragmatic movement is more important, by far. The diaphragm is the biggest single muscle in the human body, the size of one's derriere. A quarter of an inch thick, it sits at the bottom of the rib cage and fills the entire body diameter at that level, from side-to-side and front-to-back, to the spinal column.

The diaphragm is the center of the universe for voice production. Ninety percent of voice production comes from here. For those who use it well, their voice is made. For those who do not, their voice will fail.

But what does "using it" mean? A combination of two actions:

— breathing with the diaphragm: knowing how to let it drop during inhalation so an adequate supply of air is available for vibrating the vocal cords
— supporting the sound with the abdominal muscles and the opposing action of the diaphragm as it rises while air is being expelled (this ensures that the proper amount of breath for vocal production is available and that breath is

used with maximum efficiency; breathing from rib-cage expansion does not ensure this).

Voice users who fail to sing with the right amount of air and fail to manage the air supply efficiently will be forced to press their vocal cords and neck muscles and throat into the mission of making sound. A recipe for vocal disaster.

The vibrator (vocal cords)

The vocal cords are located at the level of the Adam's apple, that firm protuberance at the front of the neck about halfway down from the bottom of the chin. The Adam's apple is more prominent in men than women. It has a notch at its top, and this notch is also more prominent in men than women.

Medically, the Adam's apple is called the thyroid cartilage — coming from the Latin word *thyros*, meaning *shield-like*,

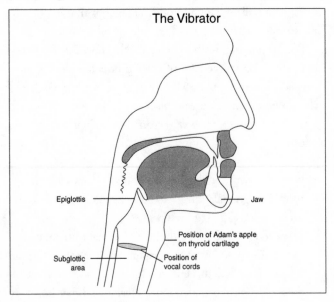

The Vibrator

Epiglottis

Jaw

Position of Adam's apple on thyroid cartilage

Subglottic area

Position of vocal cords

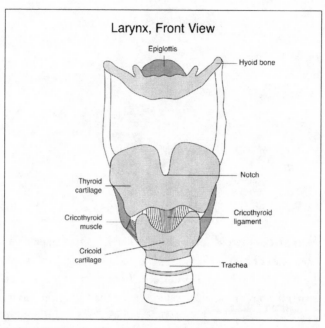

Larynx, Front View

Epiglottis

Hyoid bone

Thyroid cartilage

Notch

Cricothyroid muscle

Cricothyroid ligament

Cricoid cartilage

Trachea

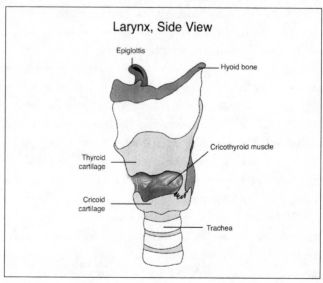

Larynx, Side View

Epiglottis

Hyoid bone

Thyroid cartilage

Cricothyroid muscle

Cricoid cartilage

Trachea

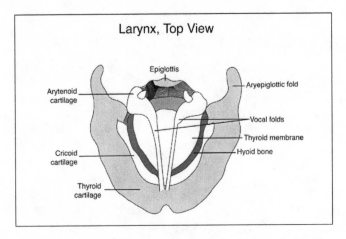

Larynx, Top View

Epiglottis

Arytenoid cartilage

Aryepiglottic fold

Vocal folds

Thyroid membrane

Cricoid cartilage

Hyoid bone

Thyroid cartilage

because the thyroid cartilage looks like a Roman shield. The metaphor of a shield is appropriate because the Adam's apple houses the larynx and protects it from injury to the vocal cords from both outside and inside. At the top of the larynx is a "trap door" that keeps fluids and food from getting into the airway. It is called the *epiglottis*, from the Latin *epi* meaning *above* and *glottis* meaning *vocal cords*.

The vocal cords are exceptionally tiny and delicate. All animals have the capacity to communicate in one way or another, but only humans have evolved to the point of having such an intricate, ingenious system. The space that houses the vocal cords and the tissues that hold them is the size of a thumbnail. The size of the vocal cords themselves is approximately the same as the white of a thumbnail. They are about 2–3 mm in thickness and about 11–17 mm long in women and 17–21 mm long in men.

The vocal cords are directly attached to the front of the thyroid cartilage, or the Adam's apple, and extend horizontally backwards in a V-shape to the back of the larynx, with the apex of the V being right behind the Adam's apple.

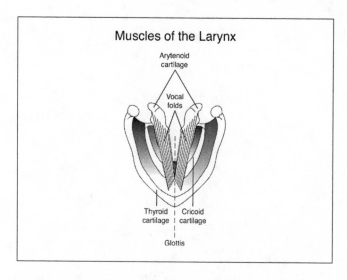

Three wisps of muscle — the thyroarytenoid, vocalis arytenoid, and the posterior cricoarytenoid muscles — are attached
to each vocal cord. These are designed to fine-tune the cords
for high notes. They are inconsequential for the vast majority
of voice users but do come into play for bel canto sopranos
and tenors, who require extra help to produce their extremely
high notes. They attach from the arytenoid cartilage that
holds the back end of the vocal cords to the front of the vocal
cords' attachment to the thyroid cartilage. These muscles pull
the cords to increase their tension and lengthen them, thus
increasing the pitch of the sound.

The resonator

The resonating space in the vocal tract is where the sound,
produced at the level of the vocal cords, is given shape. From
top to bottom, the anatomical structures involved in res-
onation are:

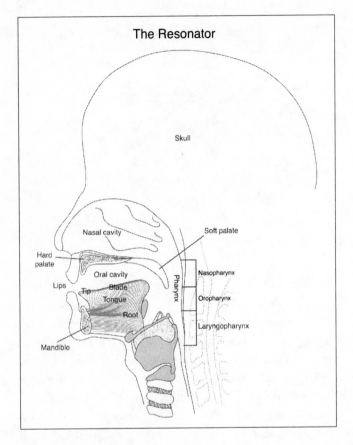

The Resonator

- the nose (nasopharynx)
- the mouth and tongue (oropharynx)
- the throat (laryngopharynx)
- and the soft palate and uvula (the back end of the soft palate that looks like a punching bag)

The resonator gives richness, quality, tone, and warmth to the sound. This is a good thing because sound produced at the level of the vocal cords is harsh and unpleasant.

The resonating space is measured from the Adam's apple to the top of the nose, where the palate is. The aim of a vocalist is to make sounds that are full, round, warm or cold, loud or soft. To do so, the vocalist must make this space as large as possible, by raising the soft palate and uvula and dropping the tongue and jaw. (This is sometimes taught to singers by telling them to get the sensation they feel at the beginning of a yawn.) The larynx itself is also dropped slightly. The bigger the space, the greater the ability to alter and shape the sound. The resonator, and how it is used, is what gives a voice its unique character.

For a person to produce a pleasing sound, each of these parts of the resonating area must be clear of swelling. For example, a person who speaks or sings while suffering a cold or sore throat will produce a tuneless sound and have little range from low to high.

The articulator

The sound, once produced, leaves the vocal tract through the articulator, which is composed of:

— the tongue
— the lips
— the cheeks
— the teeth
— and the skull and sinuses

These structures shape the sound from below into words of all languages and other vocal gestures. The articulation of vowels in combination with consonant sounds lends shape to the style or genre of music being sung. Rock singers use a tighter throat and back tongue, creating a "yeah, yeah, yeah"

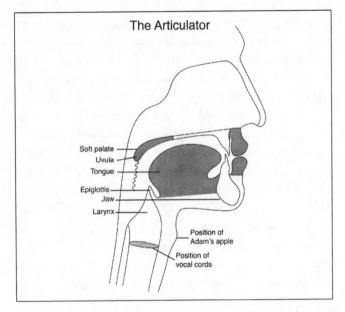

The Articulator

Soft palate
Uvula
Tongue
Epiglottis
Jaw
Larynx

Position of
Adam's apple

Position of
vocal cords

sound, whereas opera singers train for years learning how to achieve perfect placement for the "yaw" sound at all pitches. To perfect the articulation of sounds in singing, some performers work on issues such as correcting a mild lisp or a distortion in sounds such as /r/ or /l/.

The Physiology of the Vocal Tract

Now we can take a look at all of these parts of the vocal tract working together.

When a voice user takes a deep breath, the diaphragm contracts and moves down, creating the physical means for the air to enter the nose and mouth. The inhaled breath travels down the windpipe (trachea), past the vocal cords (larynx), en route to the lungs.

One can get a good sense of the proper action of the diaphragm in speaking or singing by placing one's fingers on the stomach and taking a deep breath. As air is taken in, the diaphragm contracts, pushing down and forcing abdominal contents down and outward. (This will force the fingers apart.) At the same time, the ribs expand or are pulled apart by the muscles between the ribs called the intercostal muscles (*costa* is the Latin word for *rib*; *inter* means *between*). More air is given entry to the already powerful diaphragm. This completes the inspiratory phase. Air is now sitting in the lungs.

At this point, one has three choices: exhale and take another breath, exhale and speak, or exhale and sing. Both speaking and singing are produced as exhalation blows the air in the lungs out past the vocal cords. As one exhales when singing or speaking, the diaphragm relaxes and rises up against the lungs. (This will bring the fingers back together.) The intercostal muscles relax, allowing the ribs to return to their normal position. The relaxation of the ribs and particularly the action of the diaphragm and abdominals combine to force the air out of the lungs, up the windpipe to the undersurface of the vocal folds, setting the vocal cords in motion.

Some sophisticated scientific principles come into play as the air strikes the undersurface of the vocal folds. The main one is Bernoulli's principle, which explains how the vocal folds move. As a person exhales, the stream of air from their diaphragm creates a positive pressure on the underside of the vocal cords. This results in a negative pressure on the top side of the vocal cords. The cords are thus forced apart and together again in rapid succession, creating sound. The front of each cord is fixed to the Adam's apple. The back end of each cord is attached to a cartilage that can move. This motion serves either to bring the cords together or move them apart.

Two movements take place in the vocal cords themselves when during voice production.

— First, the cords move apart and together, opening and closing in response to the air generated from the diaphragm.
— Second, each cord has its own individual movement. (More about this later.)

Together these two types of movement produce the sound wave.

The vocal cords move apart and together anywhere from 40 to more than 1,000 times per second. Each movement of the vocal cords apart and together constitutes one cycle. This rapid movement is what creates sound. The lower the number of vibrations, or cycles, of the vocal cords, the lower the sound; the higher the number, the higher the sound.

The secret of clarity or pureness of sound lies in how closely the vocal cords touch each other: how much they approximate each other, making a complete seal when they touch. To complete a full cycle and to produce a clear sound, each cord must "kiss" almost the entirety of the other cord and close. Singers with good technique allow little or no leakage of airflow when their vocal cords are touching each other.

Think of how a butcher's knife must be clean and sharp to cut meat without tearing. Similarly, for voice users to create the sound they are striving for, the column of air must be cut cleanly and sharply by the edges of the vocal cords. The more sharply the airstream is cut and the better the seal of the vocal folds when they touch each other, the purer the sound.

The secret of good vocal tone lies in how effectively the right amount of airflow is created via the generator (diaphragm) to close the folds, while keeping them moving.

So far an energy source has been created through the diaphragm to introduce the movement of air into the voice-production system. This has caused the vocal cords to vibrate, creating sound.

At this point the sound is en route to the part of the vocal tract called the vibrator. This is where the sound is formed and made tuneful.

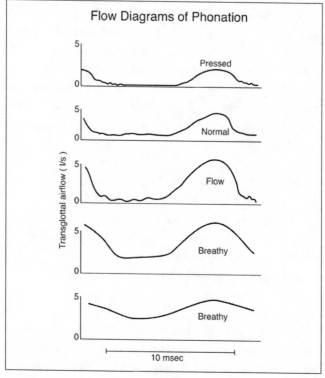

Diagrams show peak air flow for these voices.

Earlier I stressed the importance of the diaphragm as the power source, the foundation of voice production. Next in importance is the health of the vocal cords themselves. The vocal cords must be smooth and white, with a sharp edge. If they are swollen or have any swellings on them, the sound they produce will be rough.

Then comes the resonator. Its proper employment consists of raising the palate and the uvula, dropping the tongue and the jaw, and lowering the larynx. If the resonating space is not used properly, the voice will be weak and strangled and will quickly fade.

The resonating space includes not only the space that can be seen when the mouth is opened but also the jaw, tongue, and palate. (What cannot be seen is the larynx itself.) Measured at rest, the resonating space is approximately 9–10 cubic centimeters. This can be increased to 14–15 cubic centimeters when the palate and uvula are raised and the jaw, tongue, and larynx are lowered. The larynx is composed of three parts:

— The epiglottis. This is the "trapdoor" at the top of the larynx that keeps food and liquids from choking us by entering our airway when we swallow.
— The glottis. This is the space between the vocal cords.
— The sub-glottic area. This is the area beneath the vocal cords where the small cartilages hold the vocal cords from the back.

The larynx is attached to the back of the tongue. A voice user's resonating space is reduced when the tongue is raised because this causes the larynx to rise. Ideally, a voice user will drop the jaw, drop the tongue, and drop the larynx to create a maximum resonating space.

All of these movements of the palate, uvula, tongue, jaw, and larynx take place instantaneously and simultaneously as air issues from the lungs powered by the diaphragm.

Finally we come to the role of the articulator: the nose, mouth, and skull. Anything that affects the clarity of this space will affect the quality of the sound. When these articulating spaces are blocked or stuffed — as a result of a cold or allergies, for instance — the sound quality will be significantly dampened and diminished.

This can be seen by talking or singing while pinching one's nostrils together. The result is a weak, thin sound with no fullness, power, or ability to project. Similarly, congestion in the nose or the sinuses or even an increase in the size of tonsils in the throat will impair the resonance and therefore the sound. These conditions reduce or impair the size of the chamber responsible for issuing the sound.

The Importance of Energy

In my experience, most medical specialists in voice are preoccupied with the vibrating and resonating parts of the vocal tract. Because these directly involve the nose and throat, they seem to them the most important elements in making sound. Perhaps there is not enough emphasis on the fact that "in the beginning was the generator": breath support via the diaphragm. The fact is, it takes energy to speak and sing.

Western medicine itself tends to dismiss the issue of energy. Like an electrician striving to fix a machine that simply needs to be plugged into an outlet, medicine sometimes focuses on the mechanics of health while overlooking the source of health: energy.

We can avoid making that mistake, however, by taking a look at the energy systems of the body and their effects on health in general and the voice in particular. The next chapter considers the chakra-based energy centers of the body as described in Buddhism. This will enable us to understand the bioelectrical energy system that supports voice production.

CHAPTER 2

ENERGY 101

As I mentioned in the introduction to this book, I am increasingly aware of the connection between body, mind, and soul in the production of sound. Time and time again I have witnessed how voice disorders can be traced back to problems in the body more generally, and from there to emotional and spiritual problems. As one writer puts it, "... the many Eastern spiritual traditions understand illness to be a depletion of one's internal power, or spirit" (Myss, 1996:70).

In my experience, over eighty-five percent of voice problems experienced by singers and actors and other voice users, whether amateur or professional, have no basis in any obvious disease of the vocal cords. Complaints of a rough voice, pain in the throat, or pain in the neck are very common. So are complaints about throat clearing, excessive phlegm, or mucous and a cough. A sensation of a lump in the throat is frequently reported. Yet these complaints are rarely caused by an actual physical problem. Rather, they are often related in some way to stress and poor breathing, which in turn relate to anxiety, depression, and spiritual crisis. That said, I must emphasize that these complaints should always be checked by an ENT physician for differential diagnoses.

The Body as an Energy System

It frustrated me, earlier in my career, that I could not find any physical causes of these very real physical problems. However, I began to find concrete solutions for voice users as I began to understand the body's energy system from the vantage point of Eastern traditions.

Most Eastern traditions believe in a form of living energy at work in the mind, body, and spirit. Buddhist and other traditions hold that we have seven ethereal energy centers, called chakras, located from the top of the head and along the spinal column to its base. These energy centers exist in pairs because they correspond to areas along the spinal cord and the parts of the body in front of these areas. *Ethereal* means that these energy centers are ether-based: They are invisible and intangible.

In this view of the body, these centers are connected to one another through pathways, or "meridians," much like telephone lines connect telephones from house to house. One energy center can affect the next — positively or negatively — and so on. The centers have been described as working in relation to each other through a kind of psycho-physical dialogue.

The seven chakras are seen in Eastern traditions as "the building blocks of all psychophysical existence" — as "psychic centers of transformation of psychic or mental energy into spiritual energy" (Johari, 72–73).

These energy centers control all bodily and psychic activities. Each one represents a hotspot of organic activity corresponding to a vital area of the body, such as the heart, the lungs, the brain, or the throat. It is believed that we can free ourselves from tension, inhibition, and stress by focusing on the health of each of these chakra areas, thus enabling the body to perform its work more freely and effectively.

These areas must be "open" to allow the free flow of energy from one level of chakra energy to the other six. There must be an easy flow of energy up the spinal column to the top of the head, as energy is taken into the body and transmitted out of the body. As one writer puts it, "From instinctual behavior to consciously planned strategies, from emotions to artistic expression, [the] chakras are the master programs that govern our life, loves, learning, and illumination" (Judith, 4).

Dr. Andrew Curran, consultant neurologist at the Royal Liverpool Hospital, offers an interesting insight into this goal of alignment. In an interview published in the *Independent* (September 20, 2005), he said, "Reproducible studies demonstrate that being unhealthy or disharmonic is an abnormal pattern that can be unlearnt, that it is possible to get rid of blockages that prevent the body from being in harmony with itself. It seems that our digestive, cardiac and immune systems as well as our emotions and spirituality are affected."

As the chakra tradition developed, the seven areas of the body were believed to correspond to different emotions and spiritual capacities. For example, the chakra at the top of the head is seen as the spiritual energy center, and the chakra corresponding to the area of the heart is seen as the emotional center.

I do not blame readers who feel a little squeamish about calling a part of the body a chakra. Most of us brought up in Western countries have been taught to be sceptical of anything other than the mechanistic model of health. But no matter: These chakras can be thought of simply as a conceptual shorthand for addressing key locations in the dynamic living system that is the human body — locations that may be affecting the voice. It should be noted, however, that modern physiology has located, in these same seven areas, the seven major nerve ganglia coming from the spinal column that regulate the body.

These seven neuroanatomical bundles correspond to chakra energy systems that control the emotional and physical balance of the body through the parasympathetic system and return it to equilibrium. They are, from the top of the body and down: the pituitary ganglia (crown chakra), the pineal ganglia (brow chakra), the pharyngeal ganglia (throat chakra), the cardiac ganglia (heart chakra), the solar ganglia (belly chakra), the pelvic ganglia (pelvis chakra), and the sacral ganglia (root chakra).

In neurological and anatomical terms, the autonomic nervous system is the body's "thermostatic control" for safety and security. The sympathetic nervous system controls our fight or flight survival reactions, and the parasympathetic system is the regulator for creating calmness. The sympathetic nerve fibers are located along the entire length of the spinal cord with major concentrations of parasympathetic bundles located where the chakras were identified by a tradition that stretches thousands of years before Western medicine exited its "barber" years.

It is also difficult in our scientific culture to discuss "spiritual energy" and maintain our credibility. However, most of us respond instinctively to the power of a great singer. Where does that power come from? Clearly not just from the singer's technical proficiency but from an artistry that is, in effect, channeling the voice. It is emotional or spiritual energy that makes the difference between the artist who sings all the right notes but gives no excitement and one who sings the right notes *and* gives us goose bumps.

The chakras illustrate how the voice is inherently connected to the larger physical and emotional components of the body. I do not pretend to suggest, however, that the chakra system and chakra work will "cut it" with a patient who is trying to finish the last lap of a concert tour without having to cancel dates and is incredibly stressed by voice difficulties three hours before show time at the Air Canada Centre in Toronto. Therapies must be adapted to the urgency of the situation and the time limits involved, but the overall understanding of voice production, in the holistic context that I am advocating, remains constant.

I have found that amateur and professional voice users are comfortable with a holistic approach to their health that combines Western and Eastern traditions. Many of them practice yoga to some extent and have a basic understanding of the chakras. When they come to our clinic with their most prized possession — their voice, which they often call their "instrument" — they find our unconventional approach comforting and reassuring, compared with the usual medical approach that all too often sends them packing if no physical causes of their problem can be located.

It is no surprise that singers are very protective of their voice. Creative singers find true happiness when they are expressing their souls with passion in their music. When their instrument is not working, they worry that this is the end of their current performance or even their career. They are emotionally attached to what they do. Personally, I believe they have an inner soul, or *neshama* (the Hebrew word for *soul*, related to the word for *breath*): a fragile emotional and spiritual sensitivity that enables creative expression. It is what makes great artists who they are: souls who feel, touch, smell, hear, see, and express themselves and their art in a special way. Joan Baez captured this when she said, "To sing is to love and affirm, to fly and soar, to coast into the hearts of the people who listen, to tell them that life is to live, that love is there ... that beauty exists and must be hunted for and found."

Many doctors roll their eyes and mutter *artists* under their breath when a sensitive actor or singer walks into their office panicking over a sore throat or case of laryngitis. But artists come by their volatility and perhaps even neuroticism honestly.

Think about it. They take big risks out there onstage as they try to create an *ideal* sound or performance while being bedeviled by the very *real* circumstances of inadequate rehearsals, eccentric directors or conductors or accompanists, and coughing audiences. And this is not to mention hostile critics, low pay, jet lag, constantly shifting schedules, exposure to the illnesses of their fellow performers and the public, and competition for their role or position.

Here's how the great tenor Enrico Caruso put it: "Each time I sing I feel there is someone waiting to destroy me, and I must fight like a bull to hold my own. The artist who boasts he is never nervous is not an artist — he is a liar or a fool." Caruso once told a Viennese journalist, "It's natural people should expect circus tricks of me, for the promises made on my behalf are as enormous as the prices charged to hear me ... The consciousness that absolutely unprecedented things are expected of me makes me ill and I fail to do half as well as I might do otherwise."

Voice specialist Norman Punt points out that voice users who are worried about "their instrument" are not being silly.

"The larynx to the singer is what hands are to the surgeon, limbs to the dancer and eyes to the marksman" (Punt, 6).

Furthermore, *any* speaker whose voice plays an important role in their work will be concerned when they are unable to channel something fundamental about themselves through the instrument of their voice. Imagine the frustration of a newscaster whose usual mellifluous baritone voice is thin and raspy. Or of a teacher who cannot be heard all the way to the back of the classroom. Or of a politician, whose thin, wavering sound inspires voters to change parties.

Introduction to the Chakras

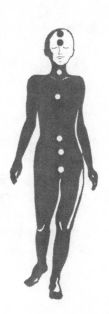

My growing understanding of the chakra energy system not only helped me personally; it also helped me professionally. I was able to show my patients how each chakra relates to the structure and function of the vocal tract and to voice production.

I will describe the chakras and their connection to vocal production in detail in the third part of this book. For now, however, let us take a quick look at each one and the important role it plays physically and spiritually in vocal production.

The seventh chakra

The seventh chakra, or crown chakra, is located just above the top of the head. In Eastern traditions, it is the *spiritual belief center*. It is present no matter how strong or how weak one's conscious spiritual belief. It symbolizes a higher power than

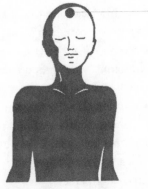

Seventh Chakra
CROWN
Spiritual Belief Center
Pituitary
Pituitary ganglia

ourselves that protects us. A number of empirical studies have shown the presence of an electromagnetic field in this and the other energy fields corresponding to the seven chakras. (Judith, 114; Myss, 1996 and 2001).

My purpose here is not to convince readers of the reality of the spiritual or the supernatural. It is to suggest that this view of things may give some credence to something that is widely believed, based on experience: that there is a central order that affects our lives. In the case of artists, something or some purpose bigger than themselves motivates them and enables them to express themselves.

For the most part, the seventh chakra speaks to truth and reality, It represents a state of consciousness that has moved beyond the duality of body and soul into a unified cosmic truth.

We will discuss this chakra in the third part of this book as "vocal spirituality."

The sixth chakra

The sixth chakra is often called the brow chakra or third eye chakra. It is located above the eyebrows, in the center of the forehead. It may be thought of as the *intuitive center*. Our intellect, intelligence, and intuitive sense are based here.

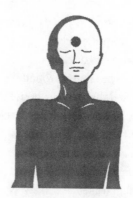

Sixth Chakra
BROW
Intuitive Center
Pineal
Pineal ganglia

This is therefore the chakra by which we judge and assess whether people are trustworthy, or whether situations are safe or unsafe.

This chakra is concerned with conscience, intellect, being, and self-realization.

We will discuss it later in the third part of this book as "vocal intuition."

The fifth chakra

The fifth chakra, or throat chakra, is located at the base of the neck. It is known as *the communication center*. This area is

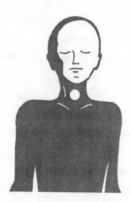

Fifth Chakra
THROAT
Communication Center
Thyroid, Parathyroid
Pharyngeal ganglia

obviously critical to voice production. It comprises the area in the neck from the Adam's apple up along the muscles of the neck, front and back, up into the jaw and ears. Located here are the muscles that surround the throat, or the pharynx, and the neck and that actually house the vocal cords. Also located here are the muscles of the shoulders, front and back of the neck, and the jaw. This area is particularly affected when a person feels stress and tension.

The throat chakra is believed to be the center of commitment, will, and judgment. It involves communication, inspiration, and expressiveness. It is adversely affected when we are carrying emotional baggage from work or home. The stress or anxiety that we feel in this area will detract from our breath support and restrict our ability to express ourselves vocally.

When this area becomes overly tense, it means that the performer is imbalanced, holding in a lot of angst or negative energy.

We will discuss this chakra in the third part of the book as "vocal communication."

The fourth chakra

The fourth chakra, or heart chakra, is represented as *the love center*. This area is concerned with forgiveness of oneself and others, emotion, and compassion. It relates to how we view ourselves and others view us. This chakra is linked to the vocalist's ability to sing with passion, heart, and artistry.

Stored here are all the hurts, pains, and emotional crises experienced from infancy to the present involving relationships with our parents, siblings, teachers, spouses, friends, employees, and employers.

These issues unconsciously cause stress. They will not necessarily be instantly resolved by chakra energy work.

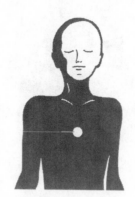

Fourth Chakra
HEART
Center of Love
Thymus
Cardiac ganglia

However, it is important for voice users to know two things in this connection: first, that tension exists in this area, and second, that blockage in this area will impede the free flow of energy in the body and adversely affect the voice.

More emphasis should be put on the practice it takes to establish a free flow of energy in breath and the body's musculature. For example, many performers feel they should focus on scales or humming in their warm-up. However, it is more important for them to assess body tension and work to release their breathing musculature, and only then to work to release tension in the voice and resonating space. In this energy work, voice users search for clarity concerning the connection between stresses or emotions, on the one hand, and past or future events, on the other. Once a person acknowledges these events, they can focus in the moment on their speaking or singing.

When the energy represented by this chakra is flowing properly, a voice user is able to communicate with greater artistry, passion, and emotion.

We will discuss this chakra later in the third part of this book as "vocal artistry."

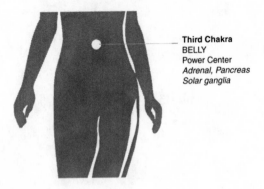

Third Chakra
BELLY
Power Center
Adrenal, Pancreas
Solar ganglia

The third chakra

The third chakra, or belly chakra, represents the *power center*. It is located in the area of the solar plexus and the diaphragm, which as already mentioned is the powerhouse of the voice. If for any reason the diaphragm cannot be accessed properly, the voice will try to support itself, generating poor-quality, inefficient sound and causing vocal damage.

This chakra expresses itself through self-love, self-confidence, and self-esteem, which it shares with the third chakra. After much experience as a doctor in general and a voice doctor in particular, and after much study of Eastern traditions, I have come to believe that weakness in this area, both metaphorically and physically, is the source of all problems involving the voice, body, and mind.

We will discuss this chakra later in the third part of this book as "vocal support."

The second chakra

The second chakra, or pelvis chakra, is the *creative center*. It is located in the pelvic area. It inspires or enables the voice user to express emotion through the voice. This is the center for expression of creativity, passion, sex, money, and power —

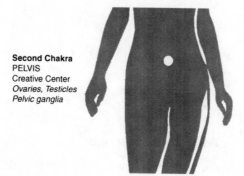

Second Chakra
PELVIS
Creative Center
Ovaries, Testicles
Pelvic ganglia

and appropriately so, because this is the physical site of sexuality and procreation.

We will discuss this chakra in the third part of this book as "vocal creativity."

The first chakra

The first chakra is often called the root chakra because it lies at the base of the spinal column. This is the *grounding center*. This chakra is the keystone of our bodies, for this is where the spine connects with the pelvis, trunk, limbs, and head: the base of the body that allows us to hold ourselves upright and

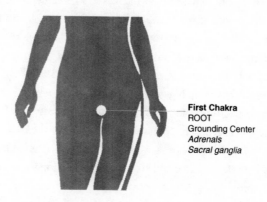

First Chakra
ROOT
Grounding Center
Adrenals
Sacral ganglia

straight. This is metaphorically the location of our moral understanding.

The first chakra is concerned with instinct, survival, and potentiality.

We will discuss this chakra in the third part of this book as "vocal stance."

The Chakras and Artistic Expression

As mentioned, for the mind, body, soul, and voice to function optimally, these seven energy centers must be open, allowing energy to flow freely from one center to the next. The Eastern view that *breathing* is what activates the chakra system is especially significant with regard to voice use, given how central good intake of breath and management of breath are, courtesy of the diaphragm and abdominal muscles.

I am aware that readers may be thinking, in the context of the description of these seven chakras, "This sounds very nice, but how does it help me understand my specific voice problem?" Take the following as an example.

A singer on tour wakes up one morning with a cold. She has shows to perform over the next ten days and she feels her cords are obviously swollen. Good technique lets her get away with it for a couple of shows but then she has a problem. The stress of not being able to count on her voice working (fifth chakra) and of letting down the rest of the musicians, the concert promoter, the record label, and the fans (fourth chakra, having to do with her emotions) has now become overwhelming. She is now complaining of a loss of range, inability to create the sound she knows she needs, and neck pain (fifth chakra); as well as of poor posture and spinal alignment (first and second chakras). She is no longer grounded (first chakra) and her inability to access her diaphragm the way she needs to (third chakra) forces her to rely for support on her throat. As a result of all this, she loses her voice.

In giving this example, which is all too common in my practice, I do not mean to suggest that voice users will necessarily be able to self-diagnose and self-treat by noticing which of the chakras are being affected in their body. The chakras are really meant to give voice users an awareness of what is happening. The benefit of having this awareness, however, can be a reduction of stress and a decrease in the tendency to panic and feel overwhelmed, in this way possibly preventing harm to the voice or hastening recovery.

The energy between chakras must be smooth and continuous up and down the body: a perfect flow in which the mind and body are totally focused on the work. There must be no blockage at any level.

For example, creative expression arises in the second (creative) chakra and is tempered by the seventh (spiritual) chakra and the fourth, or heart chakra (forgiveness, love, and emotion). Vocal expression is generated by the third chakra of self-love, self-confidence, and self-trust. It is shaped and delivered by the fifth chakra (communication).

To grasp the entire system, consider that artistic creation originates at the root of the spine, created at the pelvis, generated by the diaphragm, producing a sound — through vocal folds, articulators, and resonators — that is tempered by our minds (intuitive sense) and intellect, and our hearts (our artistic expression of love, forgiveness, and emotions).

⌒

In this and the previous chapter, we have looked at the basic structures of the voice and at vocal energy. We turn now to actual vocal problems. We will return to the chakras in the final part of the book, examining the relationship between each of them and the anatomical, physiological, and psychological aspects of voice production: the mind, body, and spirit connection involved in producing sound.

PART II

THE DISORDERED VOICE

CHAPTER 3

A VISIT TO THE VOICE DOCTOR

This chapter describes a visit to the voice doctor to familiarize readers with common vocal complaints and how they are examined.

Chapter 4 will zero in on the most common voice problem caused by misuse or abuse of the voice: muscular tension dysphonia. (*Dysphonia* is a medical term for a disturbance of the voice.) MTD is a condition in which the voice has been injured because the voice user has misguidedly used the muscles of the neck and surrounding area, instead of the diaphragm, to support and project the voice.

And chapter 5 will explore other vocal problems created by misuse and abuse of the voice.

Note that this book does not cover vocal problems caused by more serious diseases such as cancer or by neurological disorders. (For a more complete list of vocal disorders, see the

Atlas of Vocal Disorders at the end of this book.) Thankfully, these conditions are rarely the source of people's vocal difficulties. Most people experiencing voice troubles can be pretty sure that their voice is structurally normal, and that using their voice properly, as described in the previous chapters, will return them to vocal health.

Voice doctors look at four categories when it comes to diagnosis and treatment:

— *Common vocal symptoms*: what is felt and experienced with the voice.
— *Common vocal signs*: what voice doctors see or discover through clinical investigation of the voice.
— *Diagnosis*: a determination of the condition the voice user is suffering from and the causes of that condition.
— *Treatment*: how the voice user should proceed in taking care of their voice now that the cause of the problem has been discovered.

We will deal with the first two of these categories in this chapter and the latter two in the two following chapters.

Common Vocal Symptoms

When meeting a new patient, I typically start off by saying, "How are you? Why are you here? What seems to be the problem? What's happening with your voice? I have a note from your doctor about a problem you're experiencing. Why don't you tell me about it in your own words?"

If you are like the majority of my patients, you will describe your symptoms in one or more of the following ways:

— My voice is hoarse, rough, breathy, or sore.

— I can sing only a few notes or say only a few words before needing a breath.

— I cannot get my low notes (or reach my high notes).

— My voice cracks or is gravelly in my passagio, creating two sounds at once (diplophonia).

— I have to clear my throat constantly because of excessive amounts of phlegm coming down the back of my nose or throat.

— I feel as if there is a big ball or lump in my throat.

— The muscles of my neck feel strangled and squeezed.

Or you may complain of:

— a loss of power

— a loss of voice

— an acidic taste in the mouth that is altering your sound.

Common Vocal Signs

In addition to the abovementioned subjective information, objective information is important: evidence that explains either what caused the underlying problem or what has happened as a result of the presence of the problem. In other words, it is my role as a doctor — and I am often assisted in this by the speech-language pathologist with whom I work — to determine any *signs* that may be connected to your *symptoms*. Vocal signs relate to both the body in general and the voice apparatus in particular.

General body deportment and posture

Unbeknownst to you, I am by now a good way down the diagnostic path. I have already begun to detect signs that may be related to your complaint. Perhaps I have noticed that you walked in tentatively and sat down uneasily. That you are slouching in your chair, as if you have little muscle control. Or that you walked in stiffly and are sitting too straight, exerting an abnormal amount of effort for such a simple task. True, most patients will feel a certain amount of anxiety in coming into any doctor's office. But what I see when you walk in and how you speak when I ask you questions about your voice — these things are very telling.

The quality of voice when speaking

Perhaps you are speaking with what is called "vocal fry": a rough-edged sound something like a creaky gate resulting from a gap between your vocal cords as you speak. (The cords should be opening and closing together with each cord closing completely.) Or your sound may seem to be coming from the back of your throat as opposed to from your diaphragm and chest or from the front of your face.

The Clinical Process

From this point in the examination I follow the classical clinical process of the medical profession.

- I note your own description of your problem.
- I take a physical history, which includes finding out how long the problem has been present, what treatments you may have already undergone for the problem, what over-the-counter or prescription drugs you have taken to

deal with the problem, and what medicines you are on for other conditions. I will ask you to describe your daily vocal habits (the different ways you use your voice, the frequency of your voice use, the volume you use in different situations). I will ask what you do for a living, and whether your job is part-time or full-time. It is important for me to know whether you are a teacher, sales clerk, server, receptionist, and so on. I also ask you about your past health, any surgery you have had, whether you smoke and if so how much, and how much coffee, tea, and alcohol you commonly consume.

— I conduct a variety of basic and technical examinations.

The first of these examinations is very basic. You know the drill: I put a tongue depressor on your tongue and ask you to say "ah." This enables me to take a look at your tongue, mouth, and throat. I watch for such things as:

— a redness at the back of your throat
— excessive amounts of saliva
— excessive amounts of phlegm
— a gagging or coughing reflex when I simply move the tongue depressor toward your mouth or place it in your mouth gently against the tongue. Your gag reflex tells me a lot. (This is discussed in greater detail in the appendix of this book.)

Next, I will feel your neck and throat area for tightness and tenderness. I will move from the base of your neck where the windpipe is, up to the three bony structures and the muscles that lift or lower the larynx, including your Adam's apple, which is where the vocal cords are actually located. (I cannot actually feel the vocal cords, however, because they are encapsulated in the larynx, behind the Adam's apple cartilage, or the thyroid cartilage.)

I may note that you feel a tenderness in your neck. For some patients, the tenderness can extend to the flat part of their lower jaw where the teeth sit and even on up into the area around their jaw joints into their ears.

Additional technical investigations

Additional investigations are required when the history and physical examination are not enough to make an exact diagnosis. This involves special technologies to visualize the vocal apparatus when it is at rest and when it is in use. The three instruments most often used for additional investigations are:

— *A flexible nasal pharyngoscope:* This is a long tube with a fiberoptic system and a camera. I insert this through a nostril and down the back of the throat, advancing toward the larynx. Along the way I am able to check

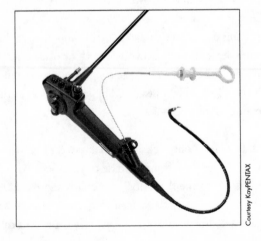

Courtesy KayPENTAX

the condition of the nose and the back of the tongue. I proceed down the back of the throat to the top of the larynx, where I can visualize the vocal cords themselves.

— *A rigid steel laryngoscope:* I use this if I need a bigger picture of the vocal cords. This device slips over the tongue and is moved to the back of the throat, hovering just above the tongue. It does not go down the throat.

— *A laryngeal videostroboscope:* This diagnostic tool adds the following to an endoscope: a continuous light and a strobe light, a video system, a TV monitor, and a computer. It allows me to record individual cycles of the vocal cords' vibrations. The strobe light illuminates the moving vocal cords intermittently. This causes the motion to appear slowed or stopped.

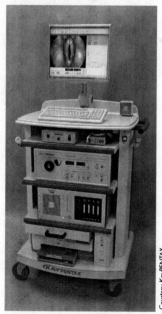

Courtesy KayPENTAX

Videostroboscope

VIDEOSTROBOSCOPY

Videostroboscopy is a procedure in which a laryngoscope with a tiny camera attached to it is inserted into the throat or nose, painlessly, visualizing on a screen the vocal folds in action. This process allows the human eye to see individual movements of the vocal folds. This is an amazing achievement when you consider (a) the size of each vocal fold — the thickness of the white of the thumbnail and less than an inch in length — and (b) the incredible speed at which the vocal folds vibrate.

To appreciate how incredible it is to record an image of the vocal folds as they vibrate, consider the fact that the human eye can record no more than 7 to 10 images on the back of the seeing mechanism of the eye, the retina, per second. (Movie pictures are made to seem seamless by giving those images at 16 or 32 or up to 70 frames per second.) And consider that the female voice, for example, vibrates at 150 to 240 cycles per second, producing those numbers of images for speaking to over 1000 cycles per second for singing.

Through videostroboscopy — adding to an endoscope a strobe light set to just under the actual vibration rate of the vocal cords — we can slow their vibrations enough to examine the individual vibration waves. This allows us to determine their ease of movement. Videostroboscopy provides information that is essential for diagnosis and treatment. The clinician can see the health of the cords as they vibrate: the color, the shape, the state of hydration, the ease of movement, the lack of movement. This technology will reveal any obvious lesion of the vocal folds, as well as the less obvious and subtle ones that routine mirror exam and regular fiberoptic examination might miss. Any abnormality of movement can be identified.

The subtle wave motion of the vocal folds — called the mucosal wave — that is intrinsic to healthy sound can also be visualized. This often proves to be a valuable teaching aid for the patient. I can show the images to the patient after explaining the workings of the voice production mechanism.

Some patients come back after successful treatment to get a "picture" of their healthy voice. This can then be given to doctors who may be dealing with them later in the various parts of the world where the singers' voice takes them. The actual recording can be copied to a CD or sent by e-mail.

Normally, the vocal cords will be a pearly white in color and will be well hydrated. They will have smooth sharp edges with no irregularities on their surface. The back of the larynx will be pink, as will the surrounding structures, which house the vocal cords.

Sometimes, however, the cords may be dry, with streaked blood vessels on the surface. The surface may be irregular because of lesions, nodules, or polyps that have formed because of continual irritation from poor technique and lifestyle conditions. The cords may be swollen. There may be puddles or globs of mucous on the cords themselves.

Typically, I will ask you to speak or sing while I examine you with one or more of these scopes. I pay special attention to the condition of the anterior third and the posterior two-thirds of the vocal cords, which, whether you have the best or worst voice in the world, is where the cords touch each other maximally with every sound produced.

I may see a swelling here, which may indicate the beginning of a polyp or nodule. These will be described in more detail in chapter 5.

The human eye can see between seven to ten movements per second. Yet the vocal cords, depending on how low or high a person is talking or singing, move between approximately 150 to 240 times per second in women and 110 to 120 times per second in men. For me to see the movement of your vocal cords more fully and accurately, I ask you to speak or talk as I examine you with an endoscope fitted with a strobe light.

How does a strobe light help me examine you better? Think back to the discotheques (dance halls) of the 1970s, which you may have experienced or at least seen in films. The strobe lights used in these halls blocked out portions of the dancers' sequential movement, causing odd visual patterns. (The lights take individual frames of people's seamless and flowing movements and black some of them out, making it look as if they are standing still and moving at the same time.)

In the 1950s, scientists began experimenting with using strobe lights to examine the vocal cords. After establishing the pitch (frequency) of the voice, they took the strobe light and applied it to the vocal cords just slower or faster than the frequency of the sound being produced. Courtesy of these scientists' pioneering work and subsequent refinement of the technologies involved, we can now watch the vocal cords in motion. We can slow the vocal cords in order to see and analyze their movement. Using this sophisticated technology, we can determine whether a patient's vocal cords are symmetrical, whether they are smooth, whether they have a sharp edge, and whether they are vibrating, or moving, equally.

Something amazing was discovered through videostroboscopy: a unique pattern of movement *within each one* of these movements of the cords as they move apart and together. This movement within the vibrations of each vocal cord is that most important phenomenon called the *mucosal wave*. We can see whether the mucosal wave is moving easily and symmetrically across each vocal cord. Each vocal cord is covered with a layer of skin, under which lies a gelatinous tissue. The mucosal wave within each vocal cord is generated within this gelatinous tissue.

The mucosal wave's movement is similar to the ripples created when a pebble is thrown into a small body of water.

These ripples move across the individual vocal cord like the ripples in a pond. The ripples are a critical feature of healthy vocal sounds. Lack of movement here can explain why a singer is having trouble reaching certain notes.

Voice doctors and speech-language pathologists and therapists are increasingly being trained to assess the sound of the voice in assessing possible vocal problems. Informally, they assess the patient's voice during their initial conversation and as they take their history. Formally, they may go on to record and analyze the patient's voice in response to various computerized acoustic tests you may have seen on *CSI*. They listen for problems with pitch, range, timbre, clarity, placement, attacks and releases, and breathing.

For example, pitch range may be checked by having the patient sing a scale as low and high as possible. Loss of range may indicate a problem with laryngeal musculature. Or if a patient reports a loss of vocal endurance, the voice doctor may test their muscle strength by having them count vigorously from one to one hundred. Breathing may be assessed as tense, shallow, or abrupt, which is what is causing the problem.

My speech-language pathologist combines information through observation, sound tests, and hands-on palpation of the neck and larynx to diagnose and rank muscular tension dysphonia.

Armed with the information gleaned from a thorough history and examination, together with information from additional testing as described, I can formulate a diagnosis. Specific voice problems are discussed in the next two chapters.

CHAPTER 4

The Most Common Vocal Problem: Muscular Tension Dysphonia

Diagnosis

Let us pick up where I left off in my examination. So far I have dealt with your symptoms and signs. I have:

— observed your body language
— listened to your voice
— taken your history and looked at your throat with a tongue depressor and palpated your neck
— used one or more scopes to observe your tongue, mouth, throat, larynx, and vocal cords.

I will most likely be able to set your mind at ease at this point, if you are like the majority of patients I see. Using a flexible fiberoptic nasoendoscope, I will show you on the monitor, as you speak or sing, that your voice is functioning properly.

And in all probability I will diagnose your problem as muscular tension dysphonia, a disorder created by:

- lack of support from the diaphragm
- a resulting inability to generate enough airflow to create sound
- and a compensatory attempt to project sound directly with the throat.

This last, ill-advised course of action creates a further problem with the resonator: It squeezes the tongue, jaw, and larynx and lifts them upward toward the throat. When voice users squeeze the muscles of the neck, they produce a squeal much like the sound a balloon makes when its neck is stretched as air is being let out. Or, too little use of the diaphragm with minimal airflow passed by the vocal folds creates a low, weak, breathy sound.

I sometimes ask singers to sing, in a glissando, from their lowest range to their highest. Many of them, instead of opening their mouth and lowering their tongue and jaw, taking in and using an appropriate amount of air, take a shallow breath and open their eyes wider and wider as if their extra air will come from the top of their head. The presence of pain in the neck muscles makes sense. Unfortunately, the pain does not stop there. The tension often causes the muscles of the neck to tighten, creating further pain. The shoulders lift upward and squeeze. The jaw tightens.

The fact that you are having trouble with your voice even though there is nothing wrong with your vocal structures will give you a certain amount of reassurance and relief. But it will also reveal certain problems with your vocal technique and practice.

For example, if you are a singer, the way you are *talking* may be causing the problem. After all, you probably actually sing only three to five percent of the time you use your voice. Talking with a lack of support from the abdominal muscles and the opposing action of the diaphragm as it rises, talking too much so the voice is not getting any rest, yelling while playing sports or at an event — these may very well be causing your singing problem.

Or you may be singing improperly, as described earlier. It is no accident that you have ended up with soreness and tension that are robbing you of your usual sound.

Much of this has to do with what I call "losing your vocal muscle memory." Let me explain.

You have probably heard of a baseball hitter who "lost his swing" or "his groove" while getting over an injury such as a strained shoulder or knee. Why does this happen? Probably because he has adopted abnormal muscle movements to compensate for tenderness or lack of function in the afflicted part of his body. Once the problem clears up, he has a new — and bad — habit. He has to relearn how to swing the bat as of old. He has to find his swing.

Similarly, singers and other voice users can "lose their voice." For example, they get a cold or a sore throat. Instead of taking time off to recover from their affliction, they work through it. In order to sing in this condition, they tense up to get something resembling normal sounds through a congested area. Eventually they get laryngitis and cannot speak or sing. Once their symptoms clear up, they have to relearn the feeling of supporting their voice with their abdominal muscles and diaphragm instead of with their neck muscles. They have to find and consolidate their vocal muscle memory. They have to get their groove back. They have to *find their voice*.

Treatments

A case from my practice illustrates one of the main treatments of muscular tension dysphonia.

A jazz singer from New York City sent me an urgent e-mail late one Wednesday evening. She was two days away from starting a three-city concert tour. She said she was unable to say a word, much less sing. A few weeks earlier she had suffered a case of sinusitis, she said. She had been treated by two doctors and put on a course of antibiotics.

I told her I would open my office for her on Thursday night. So up she flew to the Toronto Island Airport and took a ferry and then a cab to my office in midtown Toronto.

My speech-language pathologist and I were waiting for her. Sure enough, she could barely croak out a greeting. She had lost her voice.

We learned that instead of resting her voice and nursing her body back to health, she had worked through her condition, continuing a busy schedule of teaching and rehearsing.

Taking her through the examination process described earlier, we discovered no pathology in her throat or vocal cords. However, we did notice that her neck, especially on the right side, was very tender, indicating significant muscle tension.

Aaron, the speech-language pathologist with whom I work, performed a detailed massage of the specific areas in her neck and throat area to reposition her larynx for optimal voice use. (This type of massage is described in more detail in chapter 6, below.) He repositioned her hyoid bone (the bone at the top of the larynx) and Adam's apple, or thyroid cartilage (behind which the vocal cords are housed). We asked her to speak, and to her surprise, speak she did. After another thirty minutes of therapy, we asked her to sing and talk. She was amazed. Her singing voice had returned. She was definitely re-finding her voice, and just in time for her tour.

When voice users say "I have lost my voice" — whether they have lost their usual tone and range or actually cannot make a sound — they are giving a psychological representation that "I have forgotten what it is like to speak or sing with ease."

We help singers by reminding them how it feels to speak and sing properly — comfortably and efficiently. We guide them back to their muscle memory of proper voice production. We teach the feeling of what it is like to have the top two structures (soft palate and uvula) lifted and the bottom three structures (tongue, jaw, and larynx) lowered, with everything supported naturally and comfortably with the abdominal muscles and diaphragm.

It is also significant, in the case described, that the singer's voice got worse the closer she got to her tour: It was as if her "inner voice" was shutting down her "outer voice" in order to force her to get help.

To summarize, most visits to my clinic include these four steps after the initial history is taken and the problem is assessed and it has been determined that they have no serious underlying medical condition:

1) I show the patient their vocal cords.
2) I reassure them that nothing is fundamentally wrong with their voice.
3) Aaron releases and repositions their larynx, all while reinstructing the patient in breath support for proper speech and voice and guiding the patient, through visual-tactile feedback therapy, back to achieving vocal resonance.

4) We sometimes prescribe drugs for them (such as anti-inflammatories, acid reflux drugs, and occasionally antibiotics).

There is sometimes a fifth step, when we refer patients to other specialists. These may include massage therapists, chiropractors, psychologists, and psychiatrists. If we suspect a medical problem is causing their problem, we refer the patient to an internist for a complete medical evaluation.

There are times when we suggest that patients suffering from MTD:

— Rest. But not absolute rest. I do not ask them to take a vow of silence, just to pace themselves, vocally, emotionally, and physically, to break the tension that is causing their problem. Absolute voice rest is never to be advised for this condition. The sooner the location of the breath is recovered, the faster the healing. (The only time I ask a patient not to use their voice at all is if they have a hemorrhage on a vocal cord.)

— Practice simple breathing exercises. Regaining access to the diaphragm is the key to resolving MTD. Repeating the following exercises several times a day will help. Try this yourself:

- Lie on your back with several large books on your stomach. Breathe slowly, making sure the books move up with each breath.
- When you breathe, pretend that the air is heavy and it is going down naturally to below your belly button.
- Practice panting, from the diaphragm, not the throat or chest. Think of the way a dog pants. Their breathing is not located in their mouth or throat; it is coming

from their diaphragm. (Note that this exercise can cause lightheadedness when done incorrectly.)

- Exhale all of your breath through your mouth and count slowly to 5. Then inhale through your nose, slowly filling your lungs by relaxing your abdominal muscles and counting slowly to 5. Repeat.

CHAPTER 5

OTHER VOCAL PROBLEMS: THE RESULTS OF ABUSE AND MISUSE

In most cases of muscular tension dysphonia, no physical abnormalities are apparent. However, tensing the neck muscles and throat and other forms of vocal misuse and abuse over time can lead to a diseased vocal tract or vocal folds.

This chapter is about these latter conditions, which I will describe under two categories: *organic (physical) vocal problems* and *psychological (stress-induced) vocal problems*.

Organic Vocal Problems

By organic vocal problems I mean physical problems resulting from *abuse* or *misuse* of the voice. Examples of abuse include over-speaking or over-singing beyond a comfortable range. Examples of misuse include speaking or singing the wrong way. In either case, the person has injured the vocal cords and obvious disease is present. This can range (in order of serious-ness) from redness caused by inflammation to a hemorrhage (a bleed into a vocal cord) to the growth of polyps, vocal nodules, or granulomas.

Hemorrhage

A hemorrhage of the vocal cords is similar to the blood clot one gets under a fingernail after a misadventure with a hammer. Singers sometimes come to my office and tell me they experienced a sudden pain in their throat while singing the night before. It was as if something tore in their throat, they say. Just like that, their voice was no longer effective. This condition requires absolute voice rest plus or minus anti-inflammatory drugs for at least two weeks.

Polyps and nodules

A hemorrhage can sometimes progress to the point that it becomes a hemorrhagic polyp. If it is not recognized and the vocalist continues to speak or sing, the polyp can progress into a nodule.

Up to the nodule stage, the vocal cord can usually recover on its own if proper therapy is given. If the problem persists, one or a combination of rest, intensive speech therapy, proper hydration, steam, and drug therapy will often do the trick. A vigorous form of this combination may even work on nodules over a longer period of time.

To understand what a nodule is, think of the callous that often forms between thumb and first finger or on the palm of the hand during gardening. In the case of the voice, this callous, or nodule, is caused by the improper functioning of one or both cords: It is created by the rubbing or pounding of the vocal cords together. The nodule can become hard. A polyp is soft and far more innocent. It is mostly on one cord and typically will often cause a corresponding indentation on the other cord. The first polyp will fit the second one similar to how a cup fits a saucer.

Swellings can be hard or soft. We prefer soft swellings because they can be healed with dietary changes, intensive voice therapy, and sometimes medications. (For more on dietary changes, see the final chapter of this book.) Hard swellings are more difficult to heal. Some of them are amenable to speech therapy. Others, if all other therapies have failed, may have to be removed surgically.

What causes these irregularities in the vocal cords? The most common culprit is repetitive misuse or abuse of the voice resulting in the cords not touching each other properly. Or it may be caused by the cords being forced together harshly, as when a person yells, screams, or coughs. Less commonly, a virus may have attacked the surface of one cord, causing swelling that can create an improper fit of this cord with the other and causing further swelling.

In my practice we use surgery as a last resort. Not everyone takes that approach, however.

An up-and-coming tenor came to see me a month before the most important event in his career: his debut at the Metropolitan Opera in New York. We discovered that he had a polyp on one of his vocal folds.

This presented him with a dilemma. Having the polyp removed surgically would get him back to singing faster than an eight-week course of therapy. Would he have the surgery and risk damaging his voice for the long term, or miss his date and risk his career advancement in the short term?

I recommended the eight-week solution. In the end he decided for the surgery, at a voice center in the U.S. where he could be attended to more quickly. He had the operation within forty-eight hours and was back to singing three weeks later — and fortunately with no harm to his voice.

Phonosurgery is a growing speciality within medicine. Phonosurgeons are ear, nose, and throat surgeons who are highly skilled at microsurgery of the vocal cords, using nothing but microscopes and very fine instruments and occasionally lasers to repair the voice.

Granulomas

Voice users sometimes suffer from granulomas, which are irritations on the vocal cords that are larger than the lesions previously described and that do not respond to conventional therapy. They are somewhat larger and they are more difficult to heal.

Granulomas are benign lesions usually caused by prolonged misuse or abuse. They can also be caused by stomach disorders: gastrointestinal reflux diseases in which acid from the stomach pours over the walls of the larynx and damages the vocal folds. The body tries to heal this by causing chronic throat clearing, but the continued irritation creates a lesion that grows larger and will not heal. We sometimes treat granulomas with drugs for reflux diseases. Other times, if they become too large and encroach on the airway, they must be removed surgically. These cases are rare.

Psychological (Stress-induced) Voice Disorders

All of the vocal problems discussed so far are *organic* in nature — that is, they have a physical cause. In such cases we can find disease in the voice and prescribe appropriate treatment.

Some voice problems, however, are *psychological*, or *stress-induced*, which is to say no physical cause can be discerned and no disease is present. These are also called *conversion reactions* or *hysterical aphonias*: a loss of voice for psychological reasons. Some of these problems have their origin in a personal tragedy involving the patients themselves or family members, causing severe emotional pain. Some people unconsciously respond to this kind of pain by shutting down their voice, which shields them from talking about their emotional pain.

One woman I worked with lost her voice after the death of her brother. She was in severe distress because she could not afford to go to the funeral, which was in the Philippines. The loss of her voice meant she was unable to telephone her family during this stressful time. To make matters worse, at work she was reassigned from her position as a senior legal secretary to mundane tasks that did not require speaking. By the time she came to me for help, she had not spoken for four years.

She could, however, cough and clear her throat. We explained to her that anyone who can do these things can talk. We showed her that her cords were healthy and were working properly. This assessment and four sessions of speech therapy reconditioned her breathing and resonance while releasing her larynx from its hold. She even phoned her family in the Philippines from our office to talk to them, for the first time in four years. She returned to her previous job and to normal communication with family and friends. She calls us yearly to thank us.

Some people lose their voice to get sympathy. Some claim compensation from their medical insurance for this problem and "cannot afford" to be healed.

One of my patients was exposed to mould spores in her building. We involved an allergist and a respirologist in the case in order to research the effect this exposure might have on her breathing. Both reports confirmed that her lungs and her blood were not poisoned and that she was not allergic to mould. We tested her voice and confirmed that, though she was speaking in a breathy, labored manner, her vocal cords were healthy. We told her that nothing was wrong with her voice. Nevertheless, she seemed unable or unwilling to make the trek back to health.

PART III

THE ORDERED VOICE

CHAPTER 6

VOCAL COMMUNICATION: THE FIFTH CHAKRA

We turn now to the healthy, ordered voice and the seven chakras. My hope is that what follows will help voice users to heal and care for their voice so they can use it optimally.

Each chapter in this part of the book deals with one of the chakras and how it relates to the voice.

A brief word about the order in which I present them. I am of course aware that in Eastern philosophy, the mind and spiritual belief are the most important aspects of life, which is why descriptions of the chakra systems typically start with the seventh chakra, located above the top of the head, and move down the body, ending with the first chakra, located at the base of the spine.

However, because this is a book about voice, I deal with the chakras in a different order. I begin with the fifth chakra, the throat chakra, because it deals with directly with the voice. I then deal with the third chakra, the belly chakra, which deals with the diaphragm, the essential support of the voice. From there I move to the fourth, or heart, chakra, dealing with emotions, which can block the throat from the breath support it needs; the first, or root, chakra, dealing with proper stance for voice use; the second, or pelvis, chakra, dealing with creativity; the sixth, or brow, chakra, dealing with intuition; and finally the seventh, or crown, chakra, dealing with spirituality.

Although it will be useful for us to look at each energy area separately, I must stress that the overall aim is *alignment*, in several senses:

- the overarching sense of the alignment of the voice user's spirit, mind, and body
- alignment within each part of the body and the related chakra
- the alignment of everything just mentioned — which is the alignment of the chakra systems.

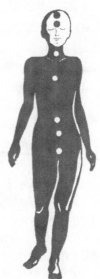

In the chakra tradition, optimal health is reached when energy flows freely from the top of the head down to the base of the spine. From the top to the bottom and the bottom to the top. Anything that affects any one of these areas will affect the others.

Let us deal in this chapter, then, with the fifth chakra, or throat chakra, which

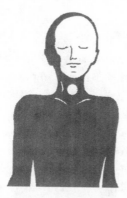

Fifth Chakra
THROAT
Communication Center
Thyroid, Parathyroid
Pharyngeal ganglia

is located in the center of the neck where the larynx is located, and behind the Adam's apple, which as mentioned earlier in the book houses the tiny white-of-the-thumbnail-sized vocal folds. This is the powerful reed that creates sound in speaking and singing.

Problems associated with this area include sore throat, stiff neck, colds, thyroid problems, and hearing problems (from referred discomfort emanating from jaw joint dysfunction).

As we have seen, tension created by forcing the voice through the throat and the neck creates most of the vocal difficulties experienced by voice users in general and singers in particular. Use of the muscles of the neck leads to throat, neck, and shoulder tension, which we call muscular tension dysphonia, the most common vocal problem. (See chapter 4.)

Patients with MTD complain of neck and shoulder tightness, excessive vocal effort, and fatigue. Muscle tightness, which can be held at the fifth chakra area through tension, stress, or misuse of the breathing mechanism, restricts the vocal folds from vibrating properly. The sound created is choked or harsh.

Similarly, failure to relax the muscles of the tongue, jaw, and the larynx and the inability to keep these structures level or sitting down will create a further pinched sound. Tension held in the larynx and the resonating space will alter voice production.

The neck muscles that surround and envelop the larynx are designed to turn the head from side-to-side, move the head forward and backward in flexing the head front and back, and move the larynx upward and downward in swallowing liquids and solids. These muscles are not designed to produce voice. When employed to do so, overuse syndrome occurs.

There are seven different inefficient muscle patterns that can create MTD. Videostroboscopy allows us to determine which one of the seven patterns is in effect and the specific type of speech-language rehabilitation that should apply.

Circumlaryngeal Massage to Reposture Anatomy

The technique most often used to treat MTD in our voice center is circumlaryngeal massage. This massage technique, developed by A.E. Aronson and modified by N. Roy, is used to assess and treat laryngeal hyperfunction. Aronson and Roy's work has shown how chronic posturing of the larynx in an elevated position leads to cramping and stiffness of the hyoid-laryngeal musculature. Aaron Low, the speech-language pathologist in my practice, was trained in this process by R.M. Shaw. Aaron has furthered this research in professionals and children. He was the first in the world to assess and treat children's voice disorders using circumlaryngeal techniques.

Manually repositioning (lowering) the larynx by kneading the circumlaryngeal area (the space between the hyoid bone and the thyroid cartilage) is thought to be the best way to reduce this tension.

In using this method of assessment and treatment, we attempt to educate the patient through an explanation of

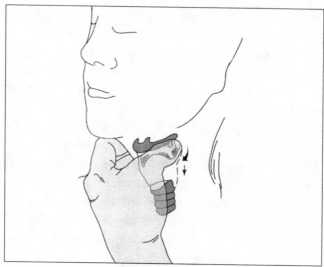

Circumlaryngeal massage

vocal anatomy and vocal physiology as well as with models and teaching aids. The teaching also emphasizes the untoward effects of excessive musculo-skeletal tension and how it causes dysphonia. This massage, performed by a skilled speech-language pathologist, takes up about twenty minutes of the initial two-hour assessment and is repeated in several weekly speech therapy sessions, to help the patient recall or create muscle memory of what it is like to speak or sing efficiently.

Important information about the correlation between the severity of laryngeal tension and a person's hoarseness can be screened and graded during the first visit. Gentle palpation of the muscles of the larynx and associated neck muscles gives us clues why a person's voice may have become hoarse or may have disappeared. Often the muscle from the base or root of the tongue lifts the hyoid bone of the larynx out of position, or the space between the hyoid bone and thyroid cartilage is closed or compressed. These muscles should be soft and allow the larynx to float freely from left to right or up and down. If tenderness or pain exists upon light touch, the voice must be released to provide the patient with the speediest possible recovery of the voice.

Laryngeal repositioning is then used in voice therapy by Aaron, along with circumlaryngeal massage and other therapy goals, to release spasms and habitual tension patterns in muscles of the larynx until normal voice is felt. The person then responds to the feeling of their voice and not the pitch or sound. Similar to how a baseball player knows, by feel and sound, that they have just hit a home run, a speaker or singer can say, "That feels right; my voice is back."

The key to this process is reconditioning the muscles back into the imprint we were born with. The muscle memory of relaxed and happy voice is always with us. However, we sometimes misplace the feeling. The goal of voice therapy is to bring it back quickly.

In the latter process, Aaron directs the patient to sense the reduction of pain and a new feeling of ease in voice production. While repositioning the larynx, he encourages the patient to vocalize (initially in their normal, everyday voice). Removing his hands, he has the patient produce this sound on their own. The key to this process is repetition, because we are helping the patient to imprint this muscle change into something called "muscle memory."

To better understand how this works, imagine that you are learning to hit a baseball for the first time. You are told numer-ous things: Stand at a right angle to the pitcher, bend your knees, bend at the waist, keep your eye on the ball, then swing by moving your weight from the front foot to the back foot. What happens? You miss the ball four or five times because you are trying to follow too many instructions all at once. Eventually, however, your body starts to simply feel how to swing and hit the ball. Your body becomes instilled with this sense of muscle memory and you rely less on your brain to remember what you are supposed to do.

This is similar to techniques used by athletes training for any sport, from gymnastics to tennis to pole-vaulting to baseball. The patient is taught to feel/envision the successful outcome of their performance and then use their voice in this free, relaxed manner.

CHAPTER 7

VOCAL SUPPORT:
THE THIRD CHAKRA

The third chakra, or belly chakra, is located in the generator, or powerhouse, of singing: the diaphragm, which is
positioned between the navel and the solar plexus. Problems
in this area include reflux esophagitis, diabetes, hypoglycemia,
and digestive difficulties.

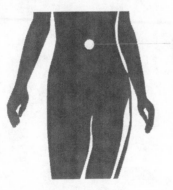

Third Chakra
BELLY
Power Center
Adrenal, Pancreas
Solar ganglia

The generator must be accessed from above through inspiration: the intake of air through the nose, mouth, and throat into the lungs. This gives voice users enough volume of airflow and hence power to vibrate the vocal cords. Voice users who speak or sing most effectively are the ones who are able to manage this column of airflow most efficiently, causing the vocal cords to seal completely as they come together during exhalation.

In Eastern tradition, the third chakra is the energy center of self-trust, self-love, will power, and self-confidence. It has been demonstrated that people do not breathe as deeply as normal when feeling insecure. Because of this, they fail to access the power of the diaphragm and thereby risk damaging their voice.

Vocalists may be anxious about a pending performance or be anxious about life in general. These emotions will almost always constrict their breathing. They do not realize that they are forgetting their training in proper breathing and supporting their sound with their diaphragm. Or they use their diaphragm properly, but *only* when they are using their voice professionally. That is, vocalists may have learned proper breathing techniques for singing or other voice use but not use them in general conversation. Anxiety can get into their speaking voice and affect their professional voice. The failure to feel self-confident manifests itself in failure to access the diaphragm for speaking, which transfers into singing. Ninety-five percent of a singer's everyday voice use is spent speaking and five percent singing. Bad speaking habits will therefore carry over to their singing voice.

I have made the point several times, but it bears repetition. It is of crucial importance for voice users to rely on the only muscle in the voice production mechanism that is capable of powering and supporting sound: the diaphragm. Count on it: If it is not relied on, all of the dysfunctional, ineffective, and inefficient compensatory aspects of voice projection in the throat will come into play.

One thing we have found is that deep breathing from the diaphragm is not sufficient for solid voice support. Proper breath support comes from a combination of *abdominal breathing* and diaphragm breathing. We encourage voice users to breathe from the abdomen as a way of helping them visualize gaining access to the diaphragm, which is so vital to healthy voice use.

Unblocking this chakra leads to proper support of the voice.

COMBINATION BREATHING

Some voice teachers talk about breathing right down to the pelvis. This is a good way to help the vocalist understand and feel what it is to breathe from their diaphragm. However, there are in fact three areas involved in breathing.

- *Clavicular breathing* is short, shallow breathing above the rib cage, at the level of the collarbone.
- *Intercostal breathing* involves the expansion and contraction of the ribs.
- *Abdominal breathing* takes place in the lower third of the abdominal wall between the hip bones.

The best breath support for speaking or singing comes from avoiding the first type of breathing and combining the second and third types.

Consider where the abdomen is and where the lower end of the rib cage is: clearly they are not the same areas. As mentioned, we use the imagery of trying to get to the abdomen because we want the voice user to access the areas below the throat and prevent themselves from tightening up. Proper vocal support comes from the combination of breathing that is slightly above the abdomen, on down to the diaphragm.

There is an important distinction between breathing from the diaphragm and supporting the voice with the diaphragm. The latter is actually a combination of support by the abdominal muscles as the diaphragm naturally rises. The great tenor Luciano Pavarotti once told an interviewer that he was breathing in with his diaphragm properly but not managing his airflow properly as he sang until he learned more about the latter when singing in an opera with the famous soprano Joan Sutherland.

- Breathing from the diaphragm — abdominal breathing — means getting optimal breath by lowering the diaphragm, below the stomach. It is more beneficial to the voice user than shallow breath in the throat or chest.
- Supporting with the diaphragm means slowly letting the diaphragm rise as one speaks or sings, letting out the exact amount of air needed for optimal phonation.

This is a useful distinction, because some voice users learn to breathe deeply but do not manage the increased air flow, letting too much out even when speaking or singing softly.

Laryngeal Release

In terms of physiology and the chakras energy system, releasing tension in the muscles of the larynx (fifth chakra) dramatically improves access to the diaphragm (third chakra). Once released, the powerful source of voice production — the diaphragm — is felt, understood, and employed. It is like the sudden surge of power felt when one steps on the gas to pass a car. This is the "aha" moment of voice production: a sudden insight into the power of the diaphragm when the muscular tension is reduced and the larynx released.

The Feldenkrais Method

Some voice practitioners and teachers use the Feldenkrais method (FM) to help their patients or students become more aware of their body generally and their breathing specifically. (It should be noted that a little learning is a dangerous thing. Voice and singing teachers are not always qualified to teach FM. Studies that lead to certification in this method are long and arduous. Anyone helping voice users through FM should be certified to do so.)

FM exercises — movement sequences — are based on the theory that improving people's observation of how they move will improve their self-awareness and enhance their self-development.

The founder, Moshe Feldenkrais, said of his method: "What I am after is more flexible minds, not just more flexible bodies."

This method fits nicely into yoga and alignment of the chakra energy systems, two traditions that aim for the unification of body, mind, and spirit.

The Alexander Technique

This technique emphasizes the "use of self." It is employed to help dancers, singers, and other performers become more aware of themselves and any internal obstructions to performance. Typically, it does not prescribe specific exercises but helps students develop new methods of achieving their goal. Ideally, this method is taught by a certified practitioner. Too often voice teachers inflict their idea of what the technique is after reading or hearing about it second hand.

Note that Alexander began as an actor and teacher and first developed his approach as a method of vocal training.

Breathing, Meditation, and the Free Flow of Energy

Breathing is central to the whole process of voice production. Breathing five to ten minutes a day in a meditative manner is a most powerful tool for voice users.

Deep breathing helps one gain access to the diaphragm and abdominal wall. Breathe deeply, seven seconds in through the nose and seven seconds out through the mouth, focusing on a sound or mantra such as "relax" — inhale a long "re-e-e"; exhale a long "l-a-x." We all know the value of this type of breathing, but what is exciting is the fact that what yogis have done for centuries, recent Western medical evidence is telling us why they have done so.

The secret is NO, nitric oxide (not nitrous oxide, or laughing gas). This gas is fleeting — it lives in our bodies for a few seconds — and creates a feeling of exhilaration, calmness, and confidence. There is a neurotransmitter in the nerve cells of many organs. It acts in the brain by causing a calming, "don't worry" effect. The gas triggers a chain reaction that allows the blood vessels to relax by releasing mood-calming chemicals.

Where is this gas found? Well, actually, the NO tank is turned on through the nose. Nitric oxide is found in highest concentration in the nasopharynx, or the back of the nose. The flow of air that occurs when we breathe through our nose on deep inhalation allows a rich source of nitric oxide to be poured into our body. The nitric oxide then helps dilate (open up) our arteries all over the body, so that the blood flows through. The source of NO is right there in our bodies, easily accessed by breathing through the nose.

We can see here how Eastern spirituality was incredibly clever and sophisticated for millennia before Western medicine caught up.

CHAPTER 8

VOCAL ARTISTRY: THE FOURTH CHAKRA

The fourth chakra, or heart chakra, is located in the area of the heart. It is the chakra associated with forgiveness, love, and emotion.

Problems in this area may include asthma, high blood pressure, and lung disease.

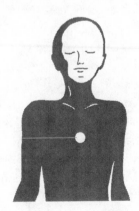

Fourth Chakra
HEART
Center of Love
Thymus
Cardiac ganglia

Underlying anxieties about life, work, health issues, and our families create angst in our minds, and angst in our minds is always manifested physically in our bodies. Our heart — our fourth chakra — over time becomes the repository of this unhappiness.

This is the dumpster bin of life. The issues here will often be resolved over time but sometimes need to be dealt with through psychotherapy.

Learning to deal with, and resolve, these anxieties is extremely important for voice users, because the anxieties can rise to the foreground and block the fifth chakra (throat) from accessing the power of the third chakra (diaphragm).

Stresses or crises held in the heart chakra weigh us down. These problems may take a great deal of time to resolve. However, voice users often experience an immediate benefit just from recognizing and accepting their stresses and understanding that they are affecting their voice.

We operate a voice clinic, not a counseling or psychiatric clinic. However, our role does involve helping voice users to recognize their stresses and "forgive" themselves for having them — that is, to accept them as a normal part of life.

The fourth chakra reveals a Catch 22 of voice production. Creative people tend to be the more sensitive than most to the difficulties of life, whether major or minor, involving relationships with parents, siblings, spouses, friends, colleagues. This sensitivity enables them to express themselves artistically, but it can also block their artistry, by denying their voice access to the diaphragm.

Sometimes singers are helped just by understanding that their emotional concerns and problems are likely to find their way into inefficient voice production. To some extent they can learn to compartmentalize their problems and their use of voice. However, in the long run they are better off personally and professionally if they deal with the emotional problems themselves, seeking professional help, if necessary. We often refer singers with fourth-chakra problems to counselors or therapists for stress reduction.

CHAPTER 9

VOCAL STANCE: THE FIRST CHAKRA

The first chakra, or root chakra, sits on either side of the sacrum: the tailbone where the bottom of the spine touches the remnant of the tail, called the coccyx.

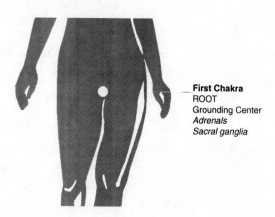

First Chakra
ROOT
Grounding Center
Adrenals
Sacral ganglia

This chakra is what holds the whole pyramid together. It holds us physically and metaphysically upward. It is the site of grounding and survival. It is the physical keystone of our bodies.

Problems in this area may include lower back pain and pain extending into the legs and buttocks (sciatica), as well as constipation and degenerative arthritis.

How does the first chakra — the base of one's spinal alignment — affect singing?

As previously mentioned, when I first meet a voice patient, I can usually determine the nature of their vocal problem by how they walk into my office, sit down in the examining chair, and begin to tell me why they are there. Their posture during any of these activities — the improper alignment of the spinal column from the shoulders to the neck to the head and down to the pelvis — alerts me to potential physical problems that can affect the voice.

Correct postural alignment is critical for efficient singing. The head sits comfortably erect on the top of the neck. The eyes are forward. The jaw is relaxed. Erect thoraco-lumbar posture with mild flexion of the hips and knees is essential for efficient access to the diaphragm and air flow. Weight should be distributed evenly to the feet.

This free flow of energy must exist from the root of the spine to the top of the head. The aim is for the voice user to feel relaxed, balanced, strong, and grounded.

Theatrical coaches and voice teachers are well advised to help their charges develop good posture. As stressed in this book, the voice needs breath support. But breath support can be obstructed by poor posture. Breathing can be obstructed, for example, if the voice user's throat is not properly aligned with their head and chest.

Voice specialists and teachers often say that to attain optimal posture for performance, the voice user should elongate their spine. This is true and should include a sense that the spine is properly aligned. Signs of poor alignment include:

— a jutting jaw
— head craned forward, or tilted downward
— rounded shoulders
— leaning to one side.

Doctors, speech-language pathologists, and voice teachers are often able to detect voice problems related to posture by sight before they hear a sound. The signs they note can include:

— increased body tension
— raising of shoulders
— elevation of one shoulder
— exaggerated use of the jaw.

It is useful to look at proper alignment from the ground up.

— Both feet should be on the floor, not too close together. Body weight should be evenly balanced on both feet.
— Legs should be straight and knees relaxed, not locked.
— The torso should be kept level, at the shoulders and the hips. The shoulders should be kept relaxed. They should not be held back or hunched forward. Shoulder blades should be released downward.
— The head should be level. This can be determined by making sure one's eyes are not looking down or up.

A good way for voice users to get a good sense of proper stance and posture for singing is to sing while standing with their heels, back, and head against a wall. Once their body is lined up properly as described above, they should continue to sing while stepping away from the wall.

Treatments for posture-related problems include regular stretching; massage therapy; chiropractic manipulation that is not too aggressive; ice on the affected area if the strain is recent and heat if not; and hot baths with appropriate aromatics such as lavender or rose, which tend to cause a calming sensation throughout the body.

CHAPTER 10

VOCAL CREATIVITY: THE SECOND CHAKRA

The second chakra, or pelvis chakra, is located in the area of the pelvis, including the lower abdomen, genitals, and womb. This energy center represents pleasure, sexuality, pro-creation, and creativity.

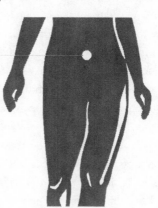

Second Chakra
PELVIS
Creative Center
Ovaries, Testicles
Pelvic ganglia

The creative source of energy from the pelvis can be blocked by emotional issues at the level of the third chakra, the diaphragm. Troubles in the heart chakra can hinder creative access to the second chakra, the pelvis, where the emotions of power, sex, money, and procreation are located. These troubles can all too easily crowd out creativity.

This area represents creativity, the area from which the performer is able to sing and express what is most important to them. The latter is transferred from the pelvis through the diaphragm (third chakra), tempered by the heart (fourth chakra), and expressed through the voice (fifth chakra).

Second-chakra energies create life; they move the earth; they make a contribution to the continuum of life. (Myss, 1996) Creative energy is physical. It is of the earth, or grounded. It is the sensation of being physically alive. This chakra generates our basic survival instincts, as well as our need to create music, art, and poetry. Our creative energy comes out of an inner tension between opposing aspects of our personality, between good and evil, forcing us to create external relationships that can resolve these conflicts.

The second chakra is one of our main resources for coping with the day-to-day events of our lives. It provides creative solutions to physical, emotional, and spiritual problems. If allowed to flow, this creative energy will reshape our life and provide more meaningful explanations for what happens in our life than we could generate with our mind alone.

People with artistic temperaments have the ability to express their passion, emotions, and sexuality through their voice.

Various types of therapists — massage therapists, craniosacral therapists, aromatherapists, and some chiropractors, for example — are able to realign energies through the various pathways from the pelvis and up the spine.

Sexual intimacy can also alleviate problems in this area. The theory in sports — and opera — used to be that sex before a performance should be avoided. Happily, this theory has been put to rest by empirical studies.

We require networks of people and relationships to help us work our way through our conflicting thoughts and emotions. This can lead us to creative study and enjoyment, guiding us to a more balanced life.

CHAPTER II

VOCAL INTUITION: THE SIXTH CHAKRA

The sixth chakra, called the brow, or third eye, chakra, is located at the center of the head, just above eye level. This chakra focuses on our seeing — inside and outside — and intuition. It is our intuitive sense, our ability to judge the safety of a situation and the trustworthiness of people.

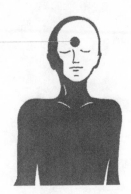

Sixth Chakra
BROW
Intuitive Center
Pineal
Pineal ganglia

Problems in this area may include loss of visual acuity, headaches, eyestrain, and blurred vision.

A lack of this kind of intuition causes uneasiness and insecurity, which can obstruct the flow of all the chakra energy systems, especially the fifth chakra, causing that problematic tension in the voice when it is out of alignment with the diaphragm, or third chakra.

The chakra energy system may be explained visualized as dominoes, with a problem in one chakra causing a problem in the one next to it, and so on, top to bottom and bottom to top.

Gifted actors, singers, and communicators in general often have an uncanny knack of connecting deeply with their audiences, somehow addressing, by the way they use their voice, their needs and aspirations. Tension at the levels of their heart and sexuality will impair this ability to connect.

It is very difficult to suggest therapies to address a lack of intuition, since it seems to fall into the category of "you have it or don't."

CHAPTER 12

VOCAL SPIRITUALITY:
THE SEVENTH CHAKRA

The seventh chakra, or crown chakra, hovers just above the top of the head. The existence of these energy lines from the place over the crown of the head and on through all of the chakras has been confirmed by physical scientific measure-

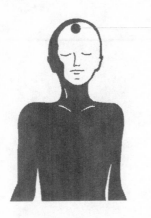

Seventh Chakra
CROWN
Spiritual Belief Center
Pituitary
Pituitary ganglia

ments. Problems in this area may include depression, alienation, confusion, boredom, and apathy.

Belief in the protective presence of God may seem unrelated to voice production. That said, most of us ascribe to a higher power, however fervently or tenuously, the ability to create — and perform — the greatest works of drama and music.

Personally, I believe that creativity is both divinely inspired and divinely given. I believe this higher power must be present in everyone in order for them to deal with each other and share with others — especially when what is being shared is a sense of beauty or artistic expression.

Whether this presence is channeled by people in terms of being a devout Christian or Muslim or Jew and whether it involves various prescriptions or proscriptions — these things are not important to me. I believe most people sense a spiritual process of some sort embedded into their beings.

Obviously people who, for whatever reason, have lost faith or hope will be blocked in their self-expression. For example, many are the cases of singers and actors who have responded to stress or depression by self-prescribing alcohol or drugs. For a time these types of spiritual substitutes may actually release creativity. But in time their ill effects on the body, mind, relationships, and employment will send the artist and the artist's gift into a downward spiral.

I believe that even the most sceptical belief in a spiritual force is enough to allow healing in this area. Simply to acknowledge some superior energy or force outside of ourselves is enough. The incredibly complex mind and body that we possess in this world and how it works almost flawlessly is proof of some guiding force that exists that cannot be fully explained by the Big Bang theory of creation.

Many performers cannot explain the power they draw upon and release but are aware that they do possess a gift to communicate beauty through their art. How can this gift be explained?

We may make distinctions between singers:

— who merely sing the notes on the page, but mechanically, in a "just the facts, ma'am" way
— who sing the right notes and also phrase the music well in accordance with the composer's intentions
— who are technically and musically sound but also bring that indefinable quality to bear on the performance: the quality that brings down the house.

I believe that the third type of singer performs from energies that come from a higher power. Singers who are open to this power, whether subconsciously or consciously, and whose energy is aligned from the top of their head to the base of their spine, in the ways described in this book, are likely not only to produce great art but to do so in a way that protects their voice and gives them, and their grateful public, a long career.

CHAPTER 13

THE WEAR, TEAR, AND CARE OF THE VOICE

I believe this book's tour of the voice will be reassuring to voice users who are experiencing any of the problems described. However, the book may prove even more helpful by helping them *prevent* these problems.

In that spirit, this conclusion gives practical pointers for the proper care of the voice.

First, think of professional athletes and how they care for themselves. It is obvious that they warm up and stretch their muscles, exercise regularly, eat nutritiously, and keep their weight at the optimal level for their particular sport.

Now think of yourself as a vocal athlete. How should you care for your voice?

Warming Up Your Voice

As a vocal athlete you should warm up your voice every day, whether you are using your voice in performance that day or not. Because, unless you are a hermit, you *will* use your voice to some extent just communicating with family, friends, and colleagues. Warming up your voice should begin with breathing exercises to release muscle tension. Warming up will help you protect it from the tensions that can creep into everyday voice use. The renowned otolaryngologist Robert Sataloff says that the failure of singers to warm up before regular voice use, not just singing, is a major cause of their vocal difficulties. "While very few singers would go out onstage to perform without having warmed up, ... many will go through an entire day of heavy voice use in classrooms, in teaching, and in other business situations without previous vocal exercise." (*Voice Foundation Newsletter*, vol. 1, no. 2, 1993)

In fact, I believe you should warm up several times a day: first thing in the morning, in the car on your way to work, before rehearsals, and before the beginning of performances.

Voice teachers generally give warm-up exercises to their singers: scales, arpeggios, and so on. I would like to make a qualification about this as a voice doctor, not a voice teacher. These exercises are fine, so long as they do not strain the voice. Each individual must first address their breathing issues before doing vocal exercises or the latter won't work. From there, tongue and lip trills and even light nasal humming are good ways to get the vocal cords into a pliable, elastic, and movable condition. Only once this condition has been achieved should the singer advance to more difficult exercises.

You could try this warm-up exercise, for instance. Hum a

pitch a little higher than your usual speaking level. Let the pitch slide slowly downward. Repeat several times. Then do the same, starting at a higher pitch. And so on.

The bottom line is, do not perform any vocal gymnastics until your breathing and voice mechanisms are ready.

Hydration

As a vocal athlete you should drink a minimum of two liters of water a day. And note that the water should be sipped, not gulped or chugged down. If you drink too much water at once, most of it will pass out through the kidneys. If you sip it, more of it will be absorbed by your body.

Why is hydration so important? Think of how oil lubricates the pistons of a car engine so they can move up and down smoothly with minimal wear and tear to the engine. Similarly, the mucous that covers your throat and larynx allows your vocal cords to move together, back and forth, and to create the mucosal wave that gives suppleness to your tone. I also tell patients to drink enough water to make their urine white (or in medical parlance, until they "pee pale").

It takes two liters of water to help the body create the three cc's of mucous needed each day to lubricate the vocal cords. Drinking the right amount of water ensures that you have enough saliva to lubricate your mouth, and enough mucous for the mucosal membrane that lubricates your throat and vocal cords.

Do not think, however, that you are getting adequate hydration by drinking tea and coffee. They are both diuretics: The caffeine they contain will make you urinate more frequently, causing you to lose water from your system. Worse, the acid that they produce in the stomach can lead to gastro-esophageal reflux disease.

Watching Your Nutritional Intake

When I use the term "diet," I am talking not so much about the number of calories you should consume daily. That is important, and so is eating balanced meals. Rather, I am talking about foods and liquids you should avoid, and particular times during which they should be avoided:

— Foods and drinks with caffeine. (See above.) These drinks dry your system. Just keep in mind that water is best. It is the elixir of vocal health. If your urine comes out yellow, you are dehydrated.

— Alcohol, which also dries out the voice. Beyond that, drinking before or after a performance is problematic in four major ways. First, alcohol is addictive. It will be all too easy for you to begin to depend on a drink to get yourself onstage. It may help you for a while, but in the end it will damage your performance. Second, alcohol engorges the blood vessels of the throat and vocal cords, which will render your tone harsh. Third, alcohol will interfere with your sleep patterns if consumed within two hours of bedtime. And fourth, alcohol taken before bedtime can cause the alcohol to rise from the stomach up to the esophagus and onto the larynx, burning the vocal folds.

— Heavy meals (pasta, tomato sauce). Eaten less than two hours before bedtime, they can cause the same problem as just described regarding alcohol.

Sleep

For you to perform well, you need good sleep, both in terms of the number of hours slept and the consistency of your sleep patterns. Many performers go to bed late and get up late, for good reasons. It is difficult for them to go to bed early and rise early on a regular basis when most of their performances are late in the evening, and when it can take several hours for their adrenaline to drop after their performance is over. This sleep pattern can work well for them as long as it is consistent.

Most people require six to eight hours of sleep a night for their body to heal and rehabilitate itself. Remember, you are a vocal athlete. Your voice needs restorative rest every bit as much as a marathon runner's muscles and cardiovascular system do.

Overall Health

You may, like many voice users, be tempted to concentrate on the health of that tiny area of the body known as the larynx and the vocal cords it houses, not concerning yourself with the rest of your body. However, as I hope this book has made clear, your entire body, mind, and soul are used when you speak or sing: You are using your body from the top of your head to the tip of your toes. Do runners exercise their legs only? What good would it be for them if their legs were strong but their cardiovascular system could not get them down the block?

Your voice will fail you if you do not support it by breathing from your diaphragm. Cardiovascular exercise is therefore important for you because it will give you greater lung capacity.

And the proper stance and posture we have discussed in this book requires strong limbs and back. Stretching exercises, moderate weightlifting, Pilates, and Core exercises can be of great help.

The Post-Performance Syndrome

If I have seen this once, I have seen it a thousand times. A singer comes to me with vocal problems — sometimes severe ones — a day or so after a performance. They are confused. Before and during the performance they were in perfect vocal shape. They warmed up properly and performed with ease. But now, seemingly out of the blue, they are experiencing strain or even loss of voice. What happened?

What happened is that they left their performance on a high and had a good time with their fellow performers at a post-performance dinner or party. They ate till late in the night, talking and laughing, having a drink or two, and inhaling second-hand smoke.

When they got up the next morning, their voice squeaked and scraped because of lack of sleep. Their throats were dry because of caffeine or alcohol intake, or from breathing in dust or smoke at the post-performance gathering. And their voices were tired because of all the talking and laughing they did the night before.

In fact, when people talk during most parties, they are actually yelling. They would realize this if the music was suddenly turned off and everyone else stopped talking. They would see that they were unconsciously raising their voice above the background noise in an effort to be heard. This can exact serious damage to the larynx and neck muscles.

It happens all too often: The efficiency of the singing voice in the performance goes seriously astray after the performance, with serious results. I am not suggesting that they become a monk or nun and avoid all celebrations after they speak or sing. But watching what they eat, drink, and breathe, avoiding excessive voice use, and getting a good night's sleep will get them back on-stage in excellent shape.

Let me wind things up with some pointers that should protect you from abusing or misusing your voice.

DO NOT ABUSE your voice

Do not clear your throat or cough habitually. *Instead:*

- sniff and swallow
- yawn to relax your throat
- swallow slowly; drink some water
- hum, concentrating on sensations of vocal resonance.

Do not yell, cheer, or scream habitually. *Instead:*

- use non-vocal sounds to attract attention: clap, whistle, ring a bell, blow a horn
- find non-vocal ways to train or discipline children and pets.

Avoid prolonged talking over long distances and outside. *Instead:*

- move closer so you can be heard without yelling
- learn good vocal projection techniques.

Avoid talking in noisy situations: over loud music, office equip-
ment, noisy classrooms, or public places, and in cars, buses,
and airplanes. *Instead:*

— reduce background noise in your daily environment
— always face the people you are talking to
— position yourself close to your listener
— wait until students or audience members are quiet and
  attentive
— find non-vocal ways to elicit attention.

Do not try to address large audiences without proper amplification. You should be able to lecture at a comfortable
loudness to be heard in any situation. *Instead:*

— use a microphone for public speaking
— learn good microphone technique.

Do not sing beyond your comfortable range. *Instead:*

— know your physical limits for pitch and loudness
— seek professional vocal training
— always use an adequate monitoring system to guide your
  voice use during performance
— never sing a high note that you cannot sing quietly.

Avoid nervous habits of public speaking that are vocally abu-
sive: throat-clearing; breath-holding; speaking quickly; speaking
on insufficient breath; speaking with a low, monotone pitch;
speaking with aggressive or low-pitched fillers (um ... ah ...).
Instead:

— ask someone to point out any vocal habits you may be unaware of
— monitor your use of these habits
— learn strategies for effective public speaking.

Do not speak extensively during strenuous physical exercise. *Instead:*

— avoid loud and aggressive vocal grunts
— after aerobic exercise, do not speak until your breathing system can accommodate optimal voice production.

DO NOT MISUSE your voice

Do not talk in a low-pitched, monotone voice. Do not allow your vocal energy to drop so low that the sound becomes rough and gravelly ("glottic fry"). *Instead:*

— keep your voice powered by breath flow, so the tone carries, varies, and rings
— allow your vocal pitch to vary as you speak.

Do not hold your breath as you are planning what to say. Avoid tense vocal onsets ("glottal attacks"). *Instead:*

— keep your throat relaxed as you begin speaking
— use breathing muscles and airflow to start speech phrases
— use coordinated voice onset.

Do not speak beyond a natural breath cycle: avoid squeezing

out the last few words of the thought with insufficient breath power. *Instead:*

➝ speak slowly, pausing often at natural phrase boundaries, so your body can breathe naturally.

Do not tighten your upper chest, shoulders, neck, and throat to breathe in, or to push sound out. *Instead:*

➝ allow your body to stay aligned and relaxed so breathing is natural
➝ allow your abdomen and rib cage to move freely.

Do not clench your teeth or tense your jaw or tongue. *Instead:*

➝ keep your upper and lower teeth separated
➝ let your jaw move freely during speech
➝ learn specific relaxation exercises.

Avoid prolonged use of unconventional vocal sounds: whispering, growls, squeaks, imitations of animal or machine noises. *Instead:*

➝ if you must talk in any such ways, use a soft vocal tone instead of a loud, harsh whisper
➝ if you must produce specific vocal effects for performance, make sure you are using a technique that minimizes muscle tension and vocal abuse.

When you sing, do not force your voice to stay in a register beyond its "flexibility limit." Flexibility must be practiced safely. Especially, do not force your chest voice too high and do not force your head voice high into falsetto range. *Instead:*

— allow vocal registers to change smoothly
— consult your singing teacher or speech-language pathologist to learn healthy techniques for smooth register transitions.

Maintain a healthy lifestyle and a healthy environment

Do not demand more of your voice than you would the rest of your body. *Instead:*

— allow for several periods of voice rest throughout the day.

Do not use your voice extensively or strenuously when you are sick or when you feel tired. *Instead:*

— rest your voice with your body: it is sick, too!

Do not use your voice when it feels strained. *Instead:*

— learn to be sensitive to the first signs of vocal fatigue: hoarseness, throat tension, dryness.

Do not ignore prolonged symptoms of vocal strain: hoarseness, throat pain, fullness, heartburn, or allergies. *Instead:*

— consult your doctor if you experience throat symptoms or voice change for more than ten days.

Do not expose your voice to excessive pollution and dehy-drating agents: cigarette smoke, chemical fumes, alcohol, caffeine, dry air. *Instead:*

— keep the air and your body clean and humid: drink 8-10 cups (2 liters) of non-caffeinated beverages daily — more if you exercise
— maintain 30% humidity in the air
— quit smoking!

Do not slouch or adopt unbalanced postures. *Instead:*

— learn and use good posture and alignment habits.

Finally, allow me to close this book by paraphrasing some lyrics from a well-known Broadway song:

Once you have found your voice — never let it go.

APPENDIX

The Gag Reflex as an Indicator of Muscular Tension Dysphonia

Over my thirty-year practice, I have seen, again and again, a marked association in my patients between a heightened gag reflex and hoarseness caused by muscular tension dysphonia (MTD). Not only that, but (a) the severity of the gag reflex seems to be a reliable indicator of the severity of MTD and (b) the gag reflex also often indicates the existence of reflux esophagitis.

This finding is significant because it means that voice care professionals other than doctors can use a simple tongue depressor to rule out, or rule in, the likelihood of MTD and/or reflux esophagitis. In severe cases, however, medical examination and advice should be sought.

To test my hypothesis of a correlation between heightened gag reflex and MTD, I conducted a two-year study of 100 professional voice users. The gag reflex was classified as follows.

Normal

A tongue depressor placed on the front third of the tongue does not stimulate tongue protrusion. The tongue sits on the floor of the mouth and the palate and uvula rise slowly and minimally. The base of the tongue and the posterior pharyngeal wall are clearly seen. (See figure 1.)

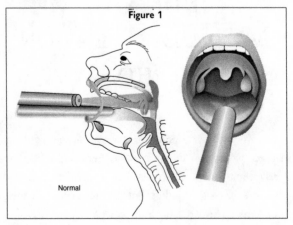

Figure 1

Normal

Grade I

With the tongue depressor in the same position as above, the back two-thirds of the tongue visibly mounds up. The oropharynx is reduced in size. The base of the tongue is no longer seen and the posterior pharyngeal is partially blocked from view. (See figure 2.)

Grade II

The tongue mounds up and exhibits tooth ridges. The palate and uvula squeeze down on the base of the

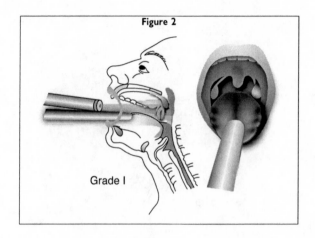

Figure 2

Grade I

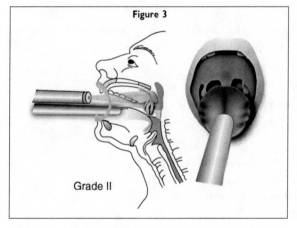

Figure 3

Grade II

tongue. The posterior pharyngeal wall is half blocked from view. (See figure 3.)

Grade III

In the most severe response, the tongue mounds up and exhibits tooth ridges as above, and the palate and uvula squeeze down on the posterior two thirds of the

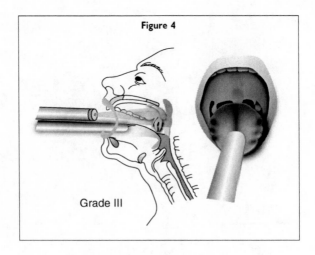

Figure 4

Grade III

tongue. The faucial pillars move medially. The posterior pharyngeal wall is now completely obscured from view. (See figure 4.)

Out of a study of 100 vocalists, the gag reflex was observed as follows:

Grade I: 46 patients (24 females, 22 males)
Grade II: 25 patients (6 females, 19 males)
Grade III: 4 patients (all female)

The remainder, 25 patients, showed a normal gag reflex.

My study confirmed a direct correlation between the severity of the gag reflex and the severity of muscular tension dysphonia as measured by the degree of muscle tightness and pain in the throat. Reflux esophagitis was also found present in nearly half of the patients. Fully 75% of the patients with muscular tension dysphonia had a heightened gag reflex, and of these, 62% also had reflux esophagitis. This was confirmed by video recording the gag reflex and by using videostroboscopy to confirm both (a) the presence of muscular tension dysphonia and its severity and (b) the presence of reflux esophagitis.

Although the connection between reflux esophagitis and muscular tension dysphonia is unclear, it has been suggested that gastroesophageal reflux may alter the motor tone of the laryngeoesophagus, consequently contributing to vocal disorders. Reducing reflux through diet, medication, therapy, and rarely surgery is likely to improve the general well being of the voice.

Patients with vocal complaints who exhibit a strong gag reflex should be examined closely by clinical endoscopy and videostroboscopy for signs of muscular tension dysphonia and reflux esophagitis.

Appendix References

Ahuja, V., M.W. Yencha, L.F. Lassen. Head and neck manifestations of gastroesophageal reflux disease. *American Family Physician* 1999: 60:873-86.

DeVault, K.R. Gastroesophageal reflux disease: extraesophageal manifestations and therapy. *Seminars in Gastrointestinal Disease* 2001; 12:46-51.

Hamdan, A.L., A.I. Sharara, A. Younes, et al. Effect of aggressive therapy on laryngeal symptoms and voice characteristics in patients with gastroesophageal reflux. *Acta Otolaryngolica* 2001; 121:868-72.

Kibblewhite, D.J. and M.D. Morrison. A double-blind controlled study of the efficacy of cimetidine in the treatment of the cervical symptoms of gastroesophageal reflux. *Journal of Otolaryngology* 1990; 19:103-9.

Koufman, J.A., J.E. Aviv, R.R. Casiano, et al. Laryngopharyngeal reflux: position statement of the committee on speech, voice, and swallowing disorders of the American Academy of Otolaryngology — Head and Neck Surgery. *Otolaryngology — Head Neck Surgery* 2002; 127:32-5.

Morrison M., L. Rammage, A.J. Emami. The irritable larynx syndrome. *Journal of Voice* 1999; 13:447-55.

Shaw, G.Y. and J.P. Searl. Laryngeal manifestations of gastroesophageal reflux before and after treatment with omeprazole. *Southern Medical Journal*, 1997; 90:1115-22.

Waring, J.P., L. Lacayo, J. Hunter, et al. Chronic cough and hoarseness in patients with severe gastroesophageal reflux disease. Diagnosis and response to therapy. *Digestive Diseases and Sciences* 1995; 40:1093-7.

Weiner, G.M., A.J. Batch and K. Radford. Dysphonia as an atypical presentation of gastro-oesophageal reflux. *Journal of Laryngology & Otology* 1995; 109:1195-6.

Wiener G.J., J.A. Koufman, W.C. Wu, et al. Chronic hoarseness secondary to gastroesophageal reflux disease: documentation with 24-h ambulatory pH monitoring. *American Journal of Gastroenterology* 1989; 84:1503-8.

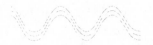

REFERENCES

Armstrong, Lance. *It's Not About the Bike: My Journey Back to Life*. New York: Putnum, 2000.

Aronson, A.E. *Clinical Voice Disorders: An Interdisciplinary Approach*. Third edition. New York: Thieme Medical Publications, 1990.

Benninger, Michael S., Barbara H. Jacobsen, and Alex F. Johnson. *Vocal Arts Medicine: The Care and Prevention of Professional Voice Disorders*. New York: Thieme Medical Publications, 1984.

Johari, Harish. *Chakras: Energy Centers of Transformation*. Revised edition. Destiny Books, 2000.

Judith, Anoden. *Wheels of Life: A User's Guide to the Chakra System*. St. Paul, MN: Llewellyn Publications, 2003.

Morrow, Nicholas H., L.A. Rammage. Diagnostic Criteria in Functional Dysphonia, *The Laryngoscope* 94, 1986: 1-8.

Myss, Caroline. *Anatomy of the Spirit: The Seven Stages of Power and Healing.* New York: Three Rivers Press, 1996.

Myss, Caroline. *Sacred Contracts: Awakening Your Divine Potential.* New York: Harmony Books, 2001.

Nair, Garyth. *The Craft of Singing.* San Diego, Oxford, Brisbane: Plural Publishing, 2007.

Philips, Pamelia S. *Singing for Dummies.* New York: Wiley Publishing, 2003.

Punt, Norman A. *The Singer's and Actor's Throat: The Vocal Mechanism of the Professional Voice User and Its Care in Health and Disease.* Third edition. London: William Heinemann Medical Books, 1979.

Roizen, Michael F. and Mehmet C. Oz, *You Staying Young: The Owner's Manual for Extending Your Warranty.* New York: Simon and Schuster, 2007.

Roy, N. and H.A. Leeper. Effects of the Manual Laryngeal Musculoskeletal Tension Reduction Technique as a Treatment for Functional Voice Disorders: Perceptual and Acoustic Measurements. *Journal of Voice* 7, 1993: 242-49.

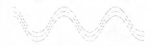

Atlas of
Vocal Disorders

Vocal problems may be most broadly categorized as:

— *Organic (physical):* caused by structural deviations of the vocal tract or disease in the vocal tract.
— *Neurologic:* caused by nerve abnormalities, affecting the muscles.
— *Psychogenic (psychological):* caused by emotional, stress-related issues. Note that these problems are often called *non-organic* (not caused by physical disease)

Organic (Physical) Vocal Disorders

angiomatous polyp: A purplish-red mass or a blood clot that can appear on the free edge of the vocal fold from sudden, harsh use of the larynx, usually resolves with absolute voice rest, medications, and, rarely, surgery.

congenital abnormalities: Developmental abnormalities of the vocal folds can affect the voice. Vocal fold paralysis and laryngomalacia are the most common. Larnygomalacia is the softening of the cartilage of the larynx structure, causing the structure to collapse and creating an alteration of voice and airway problem.

contact ulcers: Raw sores on the mucous membrane of the vocal fold. Usually caused by voice abuse.

endocrine changes: Thyroid disorders and hormonal changes may diminish voice quality.

granuloma: A lump of chronically irritated tissue, localized in the larynx. Also known as "proud flesh," it is most typically found in the back of the vocal fold, in response to an endotracheal tube used for general anaesthetic for surgical procedures or to reflux esophagitis. Almost always requires surgery.

hyperkeratosis: A horny overgrowth on the vocal folds caused by a layered build-up of thick, hard cell tissue.

infectious laryngitis: Usually indicated by inflammation of the larynx causing hoarseness or loss of voice, and almost always caused by a virus.

laryngectomy: Surgical removal of the larynx.

leukoplakia: A lesion most frequently seen on the vocal fold of chronic smokers or others with chronic inflammation. Literally, "white patch."

papilloma: A wart-like lesion, caused by a virus, on the vocal fold surface that may extend into the fold as far as the vocalis muscle. Vocal quality is usually severely dysphonic.

nodules: A hard, callous-like lesion of the vocal fold, most commonly caused by vocal misuse/abuse. Usually associated with a mirror deformity or concavity on the opposite fold (a "cup and saucer" deformity). Nodules sometimes require surgery. Most respond to speech therapy.

polyp: Benign soft swelling on the vocal cord caused by sudden, harsh use of the voice. Swelling can be filled with fluid or blood. Most commonly resolved with speech therapy and, on occasion, medications. Polyps rarely require surgery.

reflux: Irritation of the laryngeal mucosa caused by acid from the stomach coming up the esophagus and burning the vocal cords. Usually treated by diet changes, over-the-counter medication, or drugs. This usually requires lifestyle changes.

Reinke's edema: Also known as *polypoid degeneration,* this is a condition of submucosal swelling most often associated with chronic smokers with heavy voice use. In women, the voice has a masculine quality.

sulcus vocalis: A ridge or furrow running the length of the middle surface of the vocal fold membrane affecting the quality of the voice.

thickening of vocal folds: Damage to vocal folds by enlargement, possibly associated with smoking or alcohol use.

webbing: A name given to tissue bridging the front of the vocal folds causing shortness of breath and noisy breathing. Although usually present from birth, webbing can also result from vocal fold trauma or surgeries.

Neurologic Vocal Disorders

multiple sclerosis: Causes tremor of the voice.

myasthenia gravis: A neurological impairment causing muscle weakness, which may result in vocal weakness.

Parkinson's disease: Causes tremor of the voice.

spasmodic dysphonia: Involuntary movements of the muscles of the larynx interfering with speech sometimes causing the voice to drop to a whisper periodically (abductory spasmodic dysphonia) or to vary in intensity, producing choppy stuttering sounds (adductor spasmodic dysphonia).

vocal fold paralysis: Caused by an injury to the nerve pathway, this is the most common neurologic voice disorder, usually accompanied by breathiness of the voice, low pitch, and occasional diplophonia. In severe cases, breathing and swallowing may be impaired. Causes include viral infections, trauma to the nerves that supply the laryngeal muscles, e.g., during neck surgery, including thyroid surgery, blunt injury to the neck.

Functional Vocal Disorders

conversion voice disorders: Can include sudden loss of voice in the absence of any organic pathology, usually brought on by a severe emotional event.

diplophonia: double pitch phonation, caused by insufficient breath support that causes the vocal folds to close incompletely, resulting in a sound that is not pure, creating two sounds.

functional dysphonia: A hoarseness of the voice most frequently found in women where there is no apparent structural abnormality.

muscular tension dysphonia: Hoarseness or rough voice resulting from excessive activity of the muscles surrounding the voice box; symptoms include neck pain, sensation of a lump in the neck, stiffness of the neck, or soreness. MTD can be caused by vocal abuse, vocal nodules, false cord dysphonia.

(The last is caused by excessive use of the false vocal cords when vocalizing.)

nodules: Minor swellings in the vocal fold where the middle and anterior thirds of the vocal cords join. These may be caused by abuse of the voice or vibratory trauma.

polyps: Fluid-filled lesions, sometimes like blisters, on the vocal fold causing hoarseness. Probably caused by voice abuse, and rarely requiring surgery.

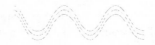

Glossary of
General Terms

abduction: Action of bringing vocal folds apart, during inhalation.

adduction: Action of bringing vocal folds together, to produce sound.

articulation: Shaping of tones by use of the tongue, lips, and jaw.

attack: Bringing the vocal folds together to create a sound. (A hard glottal attack — bringing the vocal folds together with pressure, creating a popping sound on release — can damage the voice.)

bel canto: Italian for "beautiful singing," a term used for a vocal style in the eighteenth century that emphasized purity of tone.

belting: Singing with the chest voice pushed upward; often used to describe the singing of female pop and Broadway singers.

break: Also referred to as a *crack*: a sudden shift in registration; inefficient sound.

breathy: Excessive air during speaking or singing, caused by inefficient closing of the vocal folds.

chest voice: Describes the lower notes of vocal ranges, which vibrate in the chest to create a thicker sound.

covering: Technique to maintain vocal quality and color throughout the vocal registers; done by rounding and darkening the vowels to avoid a "white" or "spread" sound.

dysphonia: Disorder resulting in poor voice quality.

edema: Swelling of the vocal folds by infection or vocal abuse.

erythema: Redness from infection or vocal abuse.

falsetto: From the Italian *falso*, used to describe the lightest and highest vocal register. Also called head *voice*.

glissando: Sliding up and down a musical scale, blurring over individual pitches.

glottal fry: Voice production that creates a popping, bubbling sound, caused by the vocal folds vibrating rhythmically but abnormally and not completely closing, sounding like a creaky door closing slowly.

glottis: The opening between the vocal folds.

harshness, hoarseness: A grating or hard quality of voice, caused by inefficient closing of the vocal folds.

head voice: See *falsetto*.

hypernasal: A resonance disorder in which too much sound comes through the nasal cavity.

hyponasal: A resonance disorder in which sounds that should come through the nasal cavity do not.

marking: A process by which a speaker or singer saves the voice during rehearsal (singing an octave lower, singing softly, saying the words in rhythm).

mask: The area where one might wear a mask - the part of the face around the nose and eyes. Used to teach the concept of placing the tone forward.

messa di voce: To crescendo and decrescendo on an individual note; used in vocal exercises to create mastery of the voice throughout the vocal registers.

passagio: Italian for *passage*; the place between registers where singers prepare for a change in registration.

phonation: Production of sound. Voice doctors and speech-language pathologists describe it various ways, e.g., as breathy, strained, or normal.

placement: The sense of positioning tones in a certain area of the body, usually the head.

projection: Production of sound to travel through space, especially in the case of singing over accompaniment.

rasp: Harsh and gravelly quality of tone.

register: Group of notes produced with similar vocal function and with similar quality of sound; registers are commonly the chest, middle, and head.

resonance: Amplification of tone determined by anatomy and the way the vocal folds and vocal tract are configured during speaking or singing. Created by maximizing the space from the top of the vocal cords to the top of the palate and uvula — raising the palate and uvula and dropping the tongue, jaw, and larynx.

respiration: The process of breathing, which in singing involves relaxing the muscles when breathing in, and supporting vocal production when breathing out.

tessitura: Italian for "texture" — the range in which most notes being sung lie.

timbre: The distinctive "color" or quality of the voice.

tremolo: Undesirable vibrato (too fast, too slow, too wide).

vibrato: Regular, even pattern of tone above and below a pitch.

videostroboscopy: Technique for visualizing the vocal cords at a rate slightly slower than their actual vibration; the illusion of slow motion allows the human eye to examine, through recorded images, the health of the vocal cords. It involves shining a flash strobe light on the vocal folds to allow them to be seen at the slow rate at which the human eye can record them.

ABOUT
BRIAN W. HANDS,
M.D., FRCS(C)

Dr. Brian Hands has sought the finest medical training available in Canada and the United States. He is a member of the Royal College of Physicians and Surgeons in his field of laryngology, sits on the Board of the Canadian Voice Foundation, is a member of the Voice Foundation in the United States, and is a member of the editorial board of *The Medical Post*. He is also a reviewer of scientific articles for *Laryngoscope* medical journal.

Dr. Hands is a voice consultant for the Canadian Opera Company, the Stratford Shakespeare Festival, the theatrical company Mirvish Productions, and major record labels.

Dr. Hands is also a landscape architect and a ceramicist.

About Vox Cura –
The Voice Specialists

Based in Toronto, Canada, Vox Cura is led by Dr. Brian W. Hands. He is joined by Aaron Low, a speech-language pathologist, and Steven Henrikson, former chair of vocal studies at the University of Windsor, in providing services that include: Ear, Nose and Throat medicine; videostroboscopy; voice rehabilitation and enhancement; speech-language pathology; voice and singing coaching; and non-traditional approaches.

Vox Cura is the only free-standing, non-hospital-affiliated voice centre in Canada and is one of the busiest medical clinics of any kind in the country.